KU-272-585

Nurse Managers
A Guide to Practice

Edited by Andrew Crowther
Foreword by Reta Creegan

AUSMED PUBLICATIONS
MELBOURNE – SAN FRANCISCO

Copyright ©Ausmed Publications Pty Ltd 2004

Ausmed Publications Pty Ltd
Melbourne – San Francisco

Melbourne office:
277 Mt Alexander Road
Ascot Vale, Melbourne, Victoria 3032, Australia
ABN 49 824 739 129
Telephone: + 61 3 9375 7311
Fax: + 61 3 9375 7299
email: <ausmed@ausmed.com.au>
website: <www.ausmed.com.au>

San Francisco office:
Martin P. Hill Consulting
870 Market Street, Suite 720
San Francisco, CA 94102
USA
Tel: 415-362-2331
Fax: 415-362-2333
Mobile: 415-309-2338
email: <mphill@pacbell.net>

Although the Publisher has taken every care to ensure the accuracy of the professional, clinical, and technical components of this publication, it accepts no responsibility for any loss or damage suffered by any person as a result of following the procedures described or acting on information set out in this publication. The Publisher reminds readers that the information in this publication is no substitute for individual medical and/or nursing assessment and treatment by professional staff.

Nurse Managers: A Guide to Practice
ISBN 0-9750445-0-8
First published by Ausmed Publications Pty Ltd, 2004.
Without limiting the rights under copyright reserved above, no part of this publication may be reproduced, stored in, or introduced into a retrieval system or transmitted in any form or by any means (electronic, mechanical, photocopying, recording, or otherwise) without the written permission of Ausmed Publications. Requests and enquiries concerning reproduction and rights should be addressed to the Publisher at the above address.

National Library of Australia Cataloguing-in-Publication data
Nurse managers : a guide to practice.

       Bibliography.
       Includes index.
       ISBN 0 9750445 0 8.

       1. Nursing services - Administration. 2. Nurse administrators.
       I. Crowther, Andrew.
       362.173068

Produced by Ginross Publishing
Book design and cover by Egan–Reid Ltd, Auckland
Cover Image: PhotoAlto
Printed in Australia

Contents

Foreword

There has never been a greater need for nurse managers at an operational level to be skilled in the technical aspects of management. Nurse managers are under increasing pressure from governments, industrial organisations, staff, and consumers of health services for greater accountability in all aspects of the nurse-management role. Taken together, these pressures create a complex management environment in which key stakeholders often have competing and conflicting priorities.

The sociopolitical environment for managers is always changing, but the fundamental principles of management have remained comparatively constant over time. Management is about managing people, and effective nurse managers need to understand both the personal context and the wider environment in which they function. A collaborative communication style based on professional respect is the first step in building a spirit of collegiality. Such a spirit of collegiality is likely to be enhanced by participative staff scheduling, fair and equitable access to learning and development, the sharing of information, performance management based on agreed objective measures, the setting of workload targets, workload distribution, the monitoring and evaluation of throughput against benchmarks, and the sharing of results and successes with staff.

Nurse Managers: A Guide to Practice is a timely and informative guide for nurse managers and those who aspire to be managers in how to manage the many situations that nurse managers are likely to encounter. A diverse range of experts with a wealth of experience brings a richness to the text. Their differing backgrounds and experience in management will be of benefit to all readers who are contemplating a career in nurse management.

Reta Creegan
RN, RM, RPN, BA Admin, FCN (NSW), FRCNA
Adjunct Professor
Centre for Health Services Management
Faculty of Nursing, Midwifery and Health
University of Technology
Sydney

Preface

Andrew Crowther

Nursing management is rapidly becoming more complex and diverse. Nurse managers are expected to have a multitude of skills apart from advanced clinical expertise. Among other tasks, they are required to understand the complexities of recruiting and rostering staff, to be able to counsel those staff, to understand the intricacies of budgeting and risk analysis, and to function as educators. In many instances, the nurse manager is underprepared for this multiplicity of roles. He or she has to 'hit the ground running', and is forced to acquire this broad range of skills almost instantly.

In addition to the expectations of nursing colleagues, nurse managers soon discover that other professions within health care have their own expectations of how the nurse manager will behave towards them, and what place the nurse manager is perceived to hold within the health-care system. In addition, there is an increasing focus around the world on efficiency and cost-cutting in health care, and governments are demanding more value for the taxpayers' money. All of these factors increase pressure on nurse managers.

Nurse Managers: A Guide to Practice is an innovative and practical text that addresses these problems, and thus fulfils a previously unmet need. The book is designed for the nurse manager in the early stages of his or her managerial career, as well as for the nurse working in a supervisory capacity for a short period of time. It offers contemporary perspectives on the variety of issues that confront the nurse manager in day-to-day practice. Beginning with an exploration of the effect that promotion has on professional relationships, and moving through such issues as leadership and motivation, the importance of moral management, dealing with unhelpful staff, occupational health and safety, and the need for an evidence-based approach to management, the reader is offered a range of solutions and coping strategies for the issues that confront nurse managers every day.

International authors from the UK, Hong Kong, Canada, Singapore, the USA, and Australia have been selected for their expertise and practical experience in their various fields. Each has contributed a concise, eminently readable chapter written in a manner that enables easy access to evidence-based information and practical advice in dealing with managerial issues as they present themselves.

The authors are aware that nurse managers practise in a variety of health-care settings, and the chapters have been prepared with this in mind. Nurse managers in acute-care hospitals, mental-health facilities, and community settings will all find that this book is of practical assistance, as will those working in remote areas, day-care settings, and facilities for the aged.

All nurses who are contemplating a career in management will find much of use in this book. The range of skills expected of nurse managers can be daunting at first, but this book provides the evidence-based information and practical advice they require to undertake their important role with growing confidence and expertise.

About the Authors

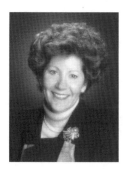

Sheila Allen
Chapter 6

Sheila Allen, who lives and practises in the United States, is a registered nurse and holds a degree in the science of nursing. She is a member of the Association of periOperative Registered Nurses (AORN), and has spoken at seminars and meetings in the USA and internationally on perioperative clinical nursing, legislative issues, bioterrorism, and professionalism. Sheila has published numerous articles in the *AORN Journal* on clinical, motivational, and organisational issues, and was editor of the publication in 2003. She currently serves as secretary for the International Federation of Perioperative Nurses and is a past president of the (US) National Association of periOperative Registered Nurses.

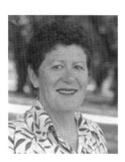

Therese Caine
Chapters 10 and 12

Therese Caine is a registered nurse who holds postgraduate qualifications in hospital administration and workplace assessment and training. Therese has had extensive experience as a nurse clinician, a health service executive, and a consultant. She has worked extensively in nursing service development, quality improvement, risk management, and change management in rural and metropolitan health services. Therese enjoys bike riding and has ridden her pushbike on long journeys from Cairns to Cape York, and from Kununurra to Broome (Australia). She is currently working in her own consultancy business using a collaborative model of work with other like-minded consultants

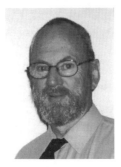

Neil Croll
Chapter 13

Neil Croll began his working life as a motor mechanic, spent some years as a research technician, and then trained as a registered psychiatric nurse at Mont Park Hospital (Victoria, Australia). He holds a degree in theology from the Melbourne College of Divinity (Victoria), graduate diplomas in community health and health administration (La Trobe University, Victoria), and a master's degree in health administration (La Trobe University). Neil has a long-standing interest in community health and reform of the health system, and is an associate fellow of the Australian College of Health Service Executives. He taught at universities before returning to the clinical field, where he now manages mental-health programs for older people as project leader, Southern Mental Health Services for Older People (Tasmania, Australia).

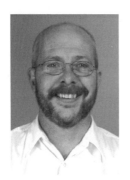

Andrew Crowther
Subject specialist editor; Chapters 7 and 21

Andrew Crowther qualified as a general and psychiatric nurse in Leicestershire (UK). His postgraduate studies include a master's degree on the subject of policy and social change (Portsmouth UK) and doctoral studies on the historical aspects of mental-hospital management (La Trobe University, Victoria, Australia). Andrew has wide experience in clinical nursing and nurse management, including a combined clinical and managerial role as coordinator of a rural community mental-health team in Australia. He has been much involved with nurse education, both in the hospital setting and in the university sector, and has taught nursing at the University of South Australia and at La Trobe University. Andrew's interests and experience in the fields of clinical nursing, nurse management, and nurse education led to his editing this important book for nurse managers. He is also the author of several mental-health nursing distance education texts and of book chapters on a variety of topics. Andrew is assistant director of nursing at the Royal Adelaide Hospital, Glenside Campus, and is an adjunct senior lecturer at the University of South Australia.

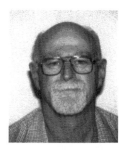

Michael Cully
Chapters 8 and 20

Michael Cully is a nurse educator at Ipswich Hospital (Queensland, Australia) with interests in mental-health nursing, care of older persons, and aggression minimisation. He has a particular interest in the mechanics of clinical decision-making under conditions of uncertainty. In his spare time, he listens to classical music, walks in the national parks of south-eastern Queensland and north-eastern New South Wales—and wonders whether the Carlton Football Club will ever win another premiership!

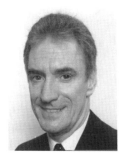

Peter French
Chapter 22

Peter French is a registered general nurse and psychiatric nurse (UK and Hong Kong) who specialises in surgical nursing and psychiatric nursing. Before moving to Hong Kong in 1991, Peter was head of the Continuing Education and Research Department at South Tees Health Authority in the UK and principal lecturer in nursing at Teesside Polytechnic UK. In his years in Hong Kong, Peter has spent time as a reader in nursing at the Chinese University of Hong Kong, chief nursing officer and principal of the Institute of Advanced Nursing Studies, and project officer for the Evidence-based Practice Project with the Hospital Authority (Hong Kong). His first degree was in social psychology and he is a chartered psychologist. Peter's doctoral degree was in education, and he has written a book on *Social Skills for Nursing Practice* and edited a book entitled *Nurse, Self & Society*. Peter has published 41 papers in refereed journals and written 20 chapters for his own and other books. He has delivered conference and guest lecturer papers in numerous countries throughout the world. Peter is currently the associate professor, School of Nursing, Hong Kong Polytechnic University.

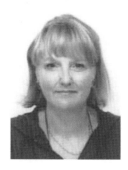

Sue Frost
Chapter 19

Professor Sue Frost is a registered nurse and nurse teacher with postgraduate qualifications in arts and education. Sue is currently dean of human and health sciences at the University of Huddersfield (UK), where she has particular expertise in the development of leadership skills in nursing. Her interest in narrative research led to a recent study of the career narratives of senior nurses in educational settings. Sue has a reputation for leading innovative developments in education, and has considerable experience in the management of change. She makes an active contribution to a range of local, national, and international developments.

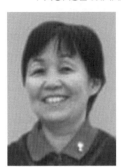

Rita Gan
Chapter 17

Rita Gan graduated in psychology from the University of Southern Queensland (Australia). She obtained a master's degree in nursing (specialising in education) from Glasgow University and a diploma in advanced nursing from Queen Margaret University College (both Scotland). Rita has had extensive experience as a staff nurse, critical-care nurse, hospital nurse manager, and university tutor and facilitator. She is currently an assistant general manager and head of education and training, Parkway Group Healthcare (Singapore). Rita has presented and published several papers on nurse management, and on professional education and training. Apart from her professional life, Rita's interests include music, reading, and travel.

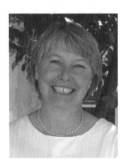

Laurie Hardingham
Chapter 3

Laurie Hardingham is the clinical ethicist at St Joseph's Health Care, London, Ontario (Canada). She has completed a fellowship in clinical ethics with the University of Toronto Joint Centre for Bioethics, and a senior fellowship in clinical ethics with the Toronto Rehabilitation Institute/University of Toronto Joint Centre for Bioethics (Canada). Laurie holds a diploma in nursing, a post-basic certificate in ICU–emergency nursing, and a bachelor's degree in nursing. She also holds an MA in philosophy from the University of Calgary (Canada). Laurie has had varied nursing experience (ICU, rural nursing, acute-care and long-term care, and nursing administration) and has taught philosophy courses for the University of Calgary and Mt Royal College. She has written a regular column 'Ethics in the Workplace' for *Alberta RN*, and has developed two *Nursing in Practice* papers for the Canadian Nurses Association, as well as having written and presented for journals, textbooks, and conferences. Her interests in bioethics include clinical ethics, end-of-life issues, gerontology, organisational ethics, and nursing ethics.

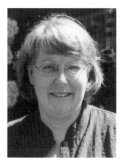

Brenda Harrison
Chapter 2

Dr Brenda Harrison operates her own independent nursing practice, Minerva Consultants, from her base in rural Victoria, Australia. She trained as a psychiatric and general nurse in the UK and has qualifications in education and management. Brenda has been a senior academic and held key clinical positions. She has also established and managed a rural community service for carers of people with mental illness. In her current practice Brenda provides management, education, and supervision, and is engaged by individuals, non-government organisations, and businesses. She also works closely with government departments and teaches periodically in Papua New Guinea

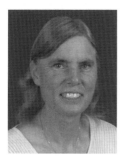

Janis Jansz
Chapter 11

Janis Jansz qualified as a registered nurse in 1969 and subsequently completed her midwifery qualifications in Western Australia (WA) and England. Janis has also completed nursing qualifications in the care of premature and sick neonates, and in coronary care. Her other nursing qualifications include a bachelor's degree in applied science, a graduate diploma in occupational safety and health, a master's degree in public health, and a doctorate of philosophy (the last from Edith Cowan University, WA). Janis has worked in a variety of city and country nursing positions. These include working as a clinical nurse in most areas of nursing, as a clinical nurse specialist for infection control, and as an area manager, nurse manager, safety adviser, nursing research coordinator, manager of quality assurance, nursing post manager, and medical centre manager. Janis currently works as a lecturer in occupational safety and health at Edith Cowan University (WA).

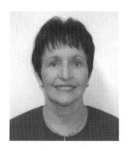

Cherrie Lowe
Chapter 16

Cherrie Lowe is a registered nurse and midwife who holds a diploma in teaching and a graduate diploma in nursing studies. Cherrie now owns and manages a successful international nursing software company, Trend Care Systems Pty Ltd, and a healthcare consulting business. This consultancy specialises in quality management and organisational efficiency. In 1999 Cherrie was awarded the Distinguished Nursing Service award by the Royal College of Nursing, Australia (Queensland).

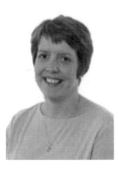

Caroline Mulcahy
Chapter 9

Caroline Mulcahy is the principal nursing officer and director of neonatal nursing services at the Royal Women's Hospital (Melbourne, Australia). Having trained as a registered nurse in London, where she also gained a graduate diploma in neonatal nursing and a master's degree in health sciences, Caroline emigrated to Australia where she undertook diverse nursing experience before becoming the unit manager of the neonatal unit of the Royal Women's Hospital. In 2000, she accepted the position of director of neonatal services at the hospital and undertook extensive reorganisation of the operational management of the unit through the application of strategic change-management techniques.

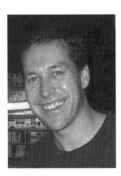

Mike Musker
Chapter 4

Mike Musker is a registered mental nurse who holds degrees in health studies and health promotion, together with diplomas in education and management. He is a member of the Institute of Healthcare Management (UK). After completing a master's degree in health at John Moores University (Liverpool, UK), Mike trained at the University of Manchester (UK) to become a registered nurse tutor. He then moved to Australia to become a senior lecturer in forensic mental health at Adelaide University and clinical manager of the Forensic Mental Health Unit of South Australia. In these roles he experiences the significant challenges of providing nurse leadership in forensic hospitals under conditions of maximum security and in situations that have the potential to attract significant media scrutiny.

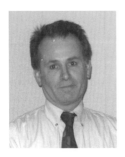

Neville Phillips
Chapter 15

Neville Phillips holds a diploma and a bachelor's degree in applied science (nursing), and a graduate diploma in adult education. He has been a nurse for nearly three decades, most of which have been spent in the field of mental health. Neville has held a range of senior management, clinical, and educational positions—including nursing director, principal nurse educator, the directorship of a metropolitan mental-health service, and clinical manager of an acute inpatient unit. For the past ten years he has been involved in various roles in a program of devolution of institutionalised services towards a mainstream community-based mental-health service in South Australia. Neville is a member of the Australian and New Zealand College of Mental Health Nurses. He is married, has two teenage daughters, and spends his spare time coaching and supporting junior sailing.

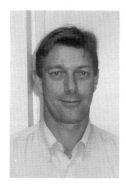

Greg Price
Chapter 14

Greg Price is a registered nurse with a diploma in nursing administration and bachelor's degree in health administration. He is a fellow of the College of Nursing and the Royal College of Nursing, Australia, and is an associate fellow of the Australian College of Health Service Executives. Since 1989 Greg has been director of nursing at the Crowley Retirement Village, Ballina (NSW, Australia)—which includes 128 self-care units. 73 community aged-care packages, and a 111-bed care centre. Greg has written numerous articles and chapters in healthcare books and journals, and has presented papers at various national conferences. In 2001 he received the Commonwealth Minister's Award for Professional Excellence in Residential Aged Care.

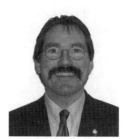

Alan Scarborough
Chapter 18

Alan Scarborough is a registered nurse and registered mental-health nurse, and a fellow of the Royal College of Nursing, Australia. Alan holds a diploma of applied science, and bachelor's and master's degrees in nursing (all Flinders University, South Australia). He also holds a master's degree in business administration (Southern Cross University, Australia). In his varied nursing career, Alan has worked as a clinician, project officer, systems manager, and senior nurse manager in a range of nursing fields, including medical and surgical, disability, and mental health. Alan has been involved in the development and implementation of information systems within Royal Adelaide Hospital (South Australia), and is committed to the provision of effective information to all levels of nursing management. He is the manager of nursing and information systems at Royal Adelaide Hospital (Glenside Campus Mental Health Service).

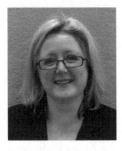

Diane Skene

Chapter 1

Diane Skene began her nursing career in 1979 and is a registered general and mental-health nurse. She holds a bachelor's degree and a diploma in nursing, and postgraduate qualifications in health counselling and child and adolescent mental-health nursing. Diane's nursing career has included positions as a clinical nurse consultant, assistant director of nursing, and service manager of child and adolescent mental health at the Monash Medical Centre (Victoria, Australia). Diane is currently acting chief operations officer at the Women's and Children's Hospital in Adelaide (South Australia).

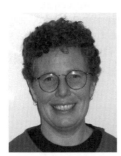

Cathie Steele

Chapters 10 and 12

Cathie Steele holds degrees in science, applied science, physiotherapy, and business. Cathie has wide experience as a clinician, manager, and a leader of change. She has worked extensively in quality improvement, risk management, change management, and strategic planning in rural and metropolitan health services. In her spare time, when she is not travelling in far-flung countries, Cathie enjoys teaching at both undergraduate and postgraduate levels and has been a guest lecturer in Australia and the UK. Her current appointment is as director of quality and patient safety at Bayside Health (Victoria, Australia).

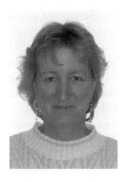

Cynthia Stuhlmiller

Chapter 5

Cynthia Stuhlmiller holds bachelor's, master's, and doctoral degrees in nursing, and is foundation chair and professor of nursing (mental health) at Flinders University (Adelaide, Australia). Her previous academic appointments include professorships and senior academic appointments in Australia, Norway, New Zealand, and the United States. Among many roles in a vast clinical background, Cynthia spent many years of pioneering work assisting Vietnam veterans with post-traumatic stress disorder and assisting disaster survivors in her volunteer work with the American Red Cross. Her research interests and publications include responses to extreme stress, disaster and emergency workers, seasonal variation, mental-health education, clinical supervision, and action-based outdoor education.

Chapter 1

The Nurse Manager

Diane Skene

Introduction

The role of the nurse manager is complex and diverse, and the nature of contemporary health care is such that a nurse manager is often hurried into the role with little time for training or preparation. A fortunate manager might have been groomed for the role by a process of succession planning, but this is not usually the case. More often there is an expectation that a new nurse manager knows what to do and how to do it without any assistance.

> 'There is an expectation that a new nurse manager knows what to do and how to do it without any assistance.'

This is patently unsafe and unacceptable—employees of a health service have a right to preparation for their roles, and employers have an obligation to supply it.

As health care diversifies, nurse managers around the world are practising in a variety of settings. Although some of the skills that are required in these various roles are detailed and specific, others form a body of shared skills and competencies common to all practice settings. Two of the most important for new nurse managers are:

▶ showing leadership; and

▶ earning respect.

Showing leadership

The terms 'manager' and 'leader' are frequently used interchangeably to describe a role of influence in orchestrating particular events. However, the terms are not synonymous. *Management* implies a meeting of goals and objectives, getting the job done, and successfully managing a range of tasks and meeting outcomes. *Leadership* is not only about meeting goals and objectives, but also encompasses *how* this is achieved. It includes such issues as how a team is developed, shaped, refined, and motivated. Leadership is thus about how management achieves its goals and objectives.

> 'Leadership is about how management achieves its goals and objectives.'

It is often asserted that 'leaders are born, not made'. According to this view, leaders are people with inherent personality traits that draw others to them, and a person either has such traits or does not. However, leadership skills *can* be learned in the same way that nursing skills can be learned. Once developed, these skills can be used to create effective leadership.

Leaders get things done in ways that support their teams. They recognise that the success of an organisation usually depends on people working together and sharing a common purpose. Leadership requires an ability to draw on the personal skills of a number of people, and to develop, refine, and implement those skills for the achievement of common goals.

Effective leaders possess two broad competencies:

▶ emotional intelligence; and

▶ strategic intelligence.

Emotional intelligence

Emotional intelligence is the ability to manage oneself and one's relationships effectively. It consists of four fundamental capacities (Goleman 2000):

▶ self-awareness;
▶ self-management;
▶ social awareness; and
▶ social skills.

Self-awareness involves understanding emotions and how they affect work performance as a manager, as well as having a realistic assessment of personal strengths and limitations.

Self-management is the ability to adjust to changing situations (and to overcome obstacles), to display honesty and integrity, and to manage responsibilities by using initiative and drive to achieve excellent personal standards and outcomes.

Social awareness is the ability to understand the needs of others and to manage colleagues by understanding their perspectives and taking an active interest in their concerns.

Social skills are the skills required to support colleagues through sensitive feedback and guidance. They include effective listening and clear concise communication, initiating new ideas, de-escalating disagreements, and creating new ways to move forward. Social skills build relationships and promote cooperation and teamwork (Goleman 2000).

Leaders with emotional intelligence are sensitive to other people's feelings. If it is necessary to criticise a staff member, nurse managers with emotional intelligence do so privately and never in front of others. They are self-aware and able to control their impatience or anger. They do not interrupt people rudely, or end conversations abruptly. Skilful application of the qualities of emotional intelligence dramatically improves teamwork and cooperation.

> 'Skilful application of the qualities of emotional intelligence dramatically improves teamwork and cooperation.'

Strategic intelligence

Strategic intelligence adds value to emotional intelligence. Strategic intelligence involves the qualities of (Maccoby 2001):

▶ foresight;
▶ systems thinking;
▶ visioning;
▶ motivating; and
▶ partnering.

Showing leadership

Effective leaders possess two broad competencies:
- emotional intelligence; and
- strategic intelligence.

Emotional intelligence

Emotional intelligence involves:
- self-awareness;
- self-management;
- social awareness; and
- social skills.

Strategic intelligence

Strategic intelligence involves:
- foresight;
- systems thinking;
- visioning;
- motivating; and
- partnering.

These topics are all explored in greater detail in the text of this chapter.

Foresight is the ability to think in terms of forces that are shaping the future. It is the ability to be aware of issues that will affect the organisation in future, and to deal with those issue through knowledge or experience.

Systems thinking is the ability to understand how elements interact, and how they fit together to make a system. System thinkers simplify essential details, and communicate these to others with clarity.

Visioning is using foresight and systems thinking to design an ideal. Visioning is not only having a picture of the future, but also directing its course.

Motivating is the ability to encourage others to embrace a common purpose and to implement a shared vision. This involves effective listening to learn what 'moves' people. Leaders who motivate are able to communicate information and a sense of meaning that inspires people to follow.

Partnering is the ability to make strategic alliances by having an awareness of the directions of the organisation and being able to manage organisational politics and build networks (Maccoby 2001).

Strategic intelligence builds upon emotional intelligence. By using both sets of competencies, a nurse manager facilitates the formation of a well-functioning team, and positions that team strategically for the present and the future.

Earning respect

Respect is not an automatic right. Rather, it is earned. To gain respect, newly appointed nurse managers need to:

- exercise self-control;
- deal effectively with requests and issues;
- value professional and individual differences;
- communicate effectively;
- address staff performance fairly;
- manage 'up, down, and sideways';
- model respect; and
- maintain clinical competence.

Each of these is discussed below.

Exercising self-control

Nurse managers are sometimes pulled in several different directions simultaneously. The manager must deal with competing emotions and keep his or her impulses under control.

It is important to 'take a breather' in stressful situations and to refrain from responding in anger or frustration. By not getting drawn into emotional situations nurse managers also model appropriate behaviour (see page 8 for more on this).

Dealing effectively with requests and issues

When it is not possible to accede to a request, it is important that nurse managers know how to 'say no'. New managers often feel that they need to agree to every request to be popular. It is important to manage time and prioritise.

Staff members might not like the fact that requests cannot be attended to straight away, and a new nurse manager might be tempted to placate impatient staff. However, rather than agreeing to a request (and then failing to deliver an outcome), respect is gained if the nurse manager is quite clear that a request cannot be met immediately—although it will be addressed later.

At the time of his or her appointment, a new nurse manager might discover that there are several issues already causing irritation to staff members—for example, complicated policies, procedures, or rules; or unrealistic performance targets. Every effort should be made to identify these issues by speaking to staff members—individually or collectively. It is a useful strategy to ask staff members to put together a list of the things that prevent them doing their jobs effectively and efficiently.

There is usually more than one issue affecting a staff group at any given time. Nurse managers should agree with staff to prioritise one issue that can be dealt with immediately, and then implement the change. Other issues can then be dealt with sequentially in a similar way. Over time staff become aware that the new manager can deal with problems efficiently and effectively. Momentum and credibility can be established in this relatively simple way.

If the manager has agreed to do something (even if he or she has second thoughts), it is essential that the agreement be followed through. Sometimes tasks take a long time to achieve—especially when there are external people involved. One way to keep the situation manageable is to update staff on current progress (for example, by putting the issues on an agenda for a staff meeting), thus ensuring that staff members know that the issue is not forgotten. Staff need to know that the nurse manager is in control and that important issues will not be forgotten.

'Staff need to know that the nurse manager is in control and that important issues will not be forgotten.'

All directions and decisions should be based on core values, and these values must be shared by staff. Organisations usually have a set of core values on which they base care practices—for example, 'partnership in care'. The nurse manager should think carefully about the practical meaning of words such as these. Nurse managers should ensure that all their actions are based on coherent and consistent policy, and that all staff members are aware of the principles guiding managerial decisions.

There might be more than one way to achieve an effective outcome. If time permits, the manager should talk with staff about alternative ways of addressing an issue. The nurse manager should be open to other people's ideas and perspectives—sometimes letting others make decisions, as long as an acceptable course of action is agreed. Shared decision-making creates a sense of responsibility and confidence in a team. This increases job satisfaction and, ultimately, has positive results for the recipients of care.

'Shared decision-making creates a sense of responsibility and confidence.'

Earning respect

To gain respect, newly appointed nurse managers need to:
- exercise self-control;
- deal effectively with requests and issues;
- value professional and individual differences;
- communicate effectively;
- address staff performance fairly;
- manage 'up, down, and sideways';
- model respect; and
- maintain clinical competence.

These topics are all explored in greater detail in the text of this chapter.

Valuing professional and individual differences

One of the roles of the nurse manager is to be above professional rivalries, and to support individual staff members according to their various skills and abilities. A nurse manager is expected to support nursing colleagues, especially in terms of their professional development. However, this must not be done at the expense of other members of the multidisciplinary team. Every discipline has particular expertise and skills that enhance organisational outcomes, and the nurse manager must ensure that these are all respected and encouraged.

Each individual member of the care team also has a different personal background, experience, and set of capabilities. An effective manager must be able to explore this range of views and collaborate product-ively. While remaining accountable for the final decision, the manager should ensure that staff members know that individual differences are valued.

> 'The manager should ensure that staff members know that individual differences are valued.'

In addition to different skills and abilities, any group of people will have a range of different understandings and opinions. If used effectively, this is a valuable resource for a manager. The nurse manager can earn respect from staff by demonstrating flexibility and the ability to accept individual differences and ideas.

Communicating effectively

The nurse manager should provide staff members with a clear understanding of how ideas and plans are progressing. Staff can then join in the vision and enhance it through collective planning. Staff members need to see that the manager has purpose and direction, and that the values underpinning the vision are synchronous with their own.

Instructions should be communicated clearly to ensure that everyone understands what is needed. To improve such communication, the nurse manager should seek feedback and encourage staff to seek clarification. However, the manager should be patient with those who need more information or additional support and direction. Other effective ways to improve clarity of communication include asking for instructions to be repeated by staff members, or following up instructions with written confirmation.

Specific praise should always be given when due. This shows that the nurse manager is keenly aware of the value of the work, ideas, and contributions of individual staff members.

Addressing staff performance fairly

If staff members fail to achieve work goals, the nurse manager needs to follow up and understand why this has occurred. In assessing a failure to meet expectations, it is important that the nurse manager reviews the validity of earlier expectations, and makes a fair assessment of any issues that might have presented a barrier to the achievement of them.

This is an important process because other staff members observe what is happening with a view to assessing the manager's ability to produce a just outcome. Staff members watch to see if the manager follows through and holds people accountable for their actions. Staff must clearly understand the organisational boundaries and performance expectations that are held by the manager.

Managing 'up, down, and sideways'

Nurse managers need to demonstrate to staff and other managers that they are willing to voice opinions in a range of forums. This helps to develop respect at all levels of the organisation, and across other organisations. Staff members need to be confident of the manager's ability to represent his or her own views—and the needs and interests of staff—at all levels and in a variety of settings.

Modelling respect

Many staff members take note of their manager's views of other senior staff. If a manager talks about other managers disrespectfully, staff members might believe that this is acceptable behaviour. In contrast, if the manager displays mature attitudes—such as flexibility, tolerance, and objectivity—this shows staff members that inappropriate behaviour or offensive statements can be dealt with in a respectful manner. Staff members are then less likely to personalise, criticise, or denigrate those who offend them.

People tend to be more comfortable around people who are similar to themselves in terms of beliefs, values, attitudes, and behaviour. Conversely, there can be a tendency to hold negative views about those who are different. All managers have staff who hold a range of beliefs, values, attitudes, and behaviours different from those of the manager. If the manager spends time with staff members in an attempt to understand their skills and motivations, these staff members are more likely to be treated as fairly

> 'A lack of fairness and consistency results in rivalry and discontent among team members.'

as any other staff members. A lack of fairness and consistency results in rivalry and discontent among team members.

Nurse managers should frequently ask for feedback when working with staff. This ensures that the manager is kept updated, and is aware of what is working well and what could be done differently. It is important that feedback is sought with a genuine desire to ascertain what is happening and with a view to acting upon it. The manager needs to be prepared for feedback that raises difficult issues. In seeking genuine feedback, and acting upon it, the manager models constructive problem-solving behaviour.

Maintaining clinical competence

New nurse managers can have difficulty finding time to remain involved in clinical activities. However, it is important to take opportunities to spend even small amounts of time in clinical work. This maintains respect and credibility, ensures that clinical skills are kept up to date, supports staff members in their work, and demonstrates that the manager is working with staff for the benefit of patients.

Conclusion

As a result of changes in the expectations of society and of the nursing profession itself, nursing has become a far more complex profession, and the need for ongoing nursing education and training has become paramount. This is particularly true of nurses who have moved into management roles. As the Royal College of Nursing, Australia, observed (RCNA 2000):

> Management preparation without clinical knowledge is an inadequate basis for managing clinical services [just as] clinical knowledge, on its own, is . . . inadequate preparation for the management role.

Given this constant state of change, the contemporary nurse manager must be a strategic planner, human-resource expert, quasi-business manager, financial analyst, risk manager, operational manager, and quality expert, as well as having an appreciation for the complexity of the clinical area (Duffield et al. 2001).

Becoming a nurse manager can be a stressful event in any nurse's career. However, it can also be a most rewarding and fulfilling opportunity.

Chapter 2

Promotion and Professional Relationships

Brenda Harrison

Introduction

As is the case in all professions, many nurses do not plan a career; rather, they let circumstances dictate professional direction and development. A career plan involves the formulating of personal and professional objectives, and the strategies thought likely to attain them. However, flexibility and frequent review of any plan are common—especially if opportunity is limited or if family and other commitments limit individual options. Despite the inherent uncertainty of a career plan, articulating a professional goal can be a powerful incentive for anyone with the determination and ability to achieve it.

> 'Articulating a professional goal can be a powerful incentive for anyone with the determination and ability to achieve it.'

Career opportunities for nurses change and develop continuously. The role of the nurse manager, however titled, is familiar world-wide. Whether the title is 'matron', 'director of nursing', 'nursing officer', 'unit manager', or 'ward sister', the essential role is to manage the work of other nurses. Not every nurse aspires to work at the most senior levels; some nurses aim to be the manager of a ward or a community area. Acknowledgment of a personal goal to be a nurse manager frequently stimulates an interest in understanding how effective managers achieve results.

Self-knowledge

One of the most effective ways of preparing for a new role involves improving self-knowledge. This can include:

▶ identifying personal strengths and weaknesses;

▶ assessing effectiveness of interpersonal communication;

▶ identifying personal and professional responses to challenging events; and

▶ accessing useful resources.

If an aspiring nurse manager is honest about personal qualities and acknowledges areas that require attention, he or she will be able to focus on personal and professional development that will enhance future career prospects. It can be helpful to consult with a trusted friend or colleague to find out whether the 'insider' and 'outsider' perspectives about self are comparable. Often the two views differ—but this might not be realised unless specific questions are asked.

Deputising for a nurse manager

It is common for clinical nurses to 'stand in' (or 'act up') for a nurse manager who is unexpectedly absent. This is usually a time-limited situation in which the established practices of the usual manager can be followed. The 'stand-in' usually focuses on the essential tasks that facilitate the day-to-day smooth operation of the area.

In many nursing workplaces a recognised position of 'associate' or 'deputy' to the ward or unit manager exists. This is an opportunity for a clinical nurse to learn about the practicalities of management using the nurse manager as role model. If they are given this sort of opportunity, many nurses discover that they enjoy managing others. Conversely, others choose not to pursue a management career because of this experience.

> 'If given a learning opportunity, many nurses discover that they enjoy managing others; others choose not to pursue a management career because of this experience.'

From clinical nurse to nurse manager

Promotion from clinical nurse to nurse manager is perceived by most nurses to be a career achievement. Some anticipatory anxiety is common. However, with thorough preparation for the role, negotiating the change from clinical nurse to nurse manager can be demanding without being personally traumatic.

Differences that new nurse managers find challenging during the period of transition from clinical nurse to nurse manager include:

▶ managing changes in working relationships with peers;
▶ spending less time working directly with patients;
▶ seeing familiar situations from a new perspective;
▶ dealing with situations not previously encountered or anticipated; and
▶ coping with situations that other nurse managers deal with effectively.
Each of these is discussed below.

Challenges for the new nurse manager

New nurse managers discover a variety of challenges as they make the transition from clinical nurse to nurse manager. These include:

• managing changes in working relationships with peers;
• spending less time working directly with patients;
• seeing familiar situations from a new perspective;
• dealing with situations not previously encountered or anticipated; and
• coping with situations that other nurse managers deal with effectively.
This list forms the framework for the text of this chapter.

Working relationships with peers

Dealing with history

Nurses who work together for a period of time get to know each other well. Common experiences, sometimes in life-and-death situations, strengthen professional and personal bonds. Individuals often share the bizarre humour that can be an integral part of coping with extreme stress or the unexpected. Features of an individual nurse's personal life can become enmeshed in the holistic relationship that develops among group members. This can be heightened if the work situation is isolated—for example, in

'Common experiences, sometimes in life-and-death situations, strengthen professional and personal bonds.'

a specialist unit, in a geographically isolated situation, or in a war zone. External pressures and experiences that nurses face together often strengthen the bonds among them.

Personal acknowledgment to nursing colleagues of the enduring value in shared experiences can signal the credibility and esteem of past relationships. Thanking others for their support and collegiality gives a clear message that, even if one is moving on, shared learning and past experiences will not be forgotten.

If a nurse from a group moves into a different role, this changes the group dynamic. Each member of the group deals with change differently. Shared experiences from the past cannot be erased—although memories of them alter with time. Some collegial friendships formed during stressful or focused periods of work last a life-time, and nurses can continue to grieve for the comfort and familiarity of past relationships—even though they might otherwise see their promotion out of the group as an exciting challenge.

> 'Nurses can continue to grieve for the comfort and familiarity of past relationships.'

Those who remain in the group can also experience difficulties. The promotion of a colleague cannot always be accepted quickly. It can take weeks or months for changes in professional roles to be generally accepted and for a new comfortable working relationship to be re-established. In addition, apart from losing familiar collegial relationships, personal professional disappointment can be a factor. If one person becomes a manager and another does not, the resentment of the person who failed to receive promotion cannot always be overcome by the new nurse manager. It might be almost impossible to overcome such disappointment, and the amount of energy expended on trying to recover a previous comfortable professional relationship should be carefully considered against the importance of devoting energy to mastering a new role.

Dividing personal and professional

Apart from testing *professional* relationships, *personal* relationships can also be tested if one person moves away from an established nursing group in which the workplace status of all members is similar. A colleague's response to a new nurse manager's promotion and

> 'Apart from testing *professional* relationships, *personal* relationships can also be tested.'

the future of any personal friendship is dependent on how well the boundaries of the personal and professional elements of the relationship have been defined in the past.

Differentiation between the personal and professional aspects of relationships with nursing colleagues can become clearer by assessing the factors listed in the Box below.

Personal or professional?

It can be difficult to differentiate between personal and professional issues in any workplace relationship. In assessing this matter, the following matters provide guidance in assessing the professional and personal aspects of a relationship:
- how often the group (or individuals from the group) meet outside work;
- the topics that dominate conversation outside work;
- the degree to which families socialise together; and
- common interests.

Moving into a nurse manager position is not a time to terminate valuable personal friendships with nursing colleagues. However, as a manager, it might become necessary to appraise, discipline, or reassign a former colleague who is also a friend. Such situations can be difficult, and they require careful planning. If the boundaries between personal and professional relationships are clear,

'If the boundaries between personal and professional relationships are clear, personal friendships are less likely to be affected.'

personal friendships are less likely to be affected. Use of tact and respect when dealing with such sensitive situations can help everyone to maintain his or her dignity.

Less time working directly with patients

Clinical nursing practice involves the provision of ongoing care to individuals and families, and sustained day-to-day contact with individuals and families is a distinctive element of nursing practice. For many nurses, the special relationships developed with patients and those close to them are central to their work, and all other aspects of work are a function of those relationships. The emotional journey in any clinical nurse's day is punctuated by conversations, shared jokes, the relief that comes with improvement, and the devastation that can accompany a patient's deterioration or death.

The importance of relationships with patients can become most evident when a nurse moves from clinical work into management. Although a role involving less direct patient care can be a relief for some newly appointed nurse managers, others have difficulty coping with less patient contact. Such nurses continue to set aside some time in their working day for direct patient care.

Fortunately, many patients and families learn quickly to consult clinical nurses on some matters, and nurse managers about others. They often help new managers to focus on their role, effectively redefining for managers a new and rewarding type of relationship with patients and their families.

If they are to plan staff rosters to maximum effect, nurse managers require a clear understanding of the knowledge and skills nurses need, and the time it takes to provide quality care. In supervising and coordinating the care that other nurses provide, nurse managers need to maintain their own clinical skills and combine this with their experience of clinical requirements and expertise.

Familiar situations from a new perspective
From the inside looking out

Promotion to the post of nurse manager does not magically transform anyone. Even with good intentions to change entrenched habits, personality traits remain relatively constant. The person who existed before a promotion is the same person who is the new nurse manager.

The organisation establishes its expectations for the work of a nurse manager through the job description, and employers and colleagues develop assumptions about how nurse managers will respond to frequently encountered situations. However, nurses in clinical and management positions often view similar situations from different perspectives. For example, a clinical nurse might use disposable equipment according to the manufacturer's instructions—reordering supplies when stocks are low. In contrast, a nurse manager is expected to identify excessive equipment usage as part of the budgetary process. This could include querying the use of certain disposable items and counselling

> 'Promotion to the post of nurse manager does not magically transform anyone . . . The person who existed before a promotion is the same person who is the new nurse manager.'

clinical nurses on how usage could be reduced without compromising patient safety or quality of care.

The responsibilities of a nurse manager involve discovering new ways to think about and deal with familiar processes and situations. Some individuals adapt to the new perspective easily, whereas others have difficulty. It can take time to grow into a nurse manager's role. The required change of focus might challenge previously held beliefs and values—including some that might not have been clearly defined or articulated. This can be confusing and confronting to new nurse managers who are forced to wrestle with what seems to be a competition between individual patient care and organisational needs. By acknowledging these conflicts, and talking with others about them, new nurse managers often find others who have encountered similar dilemmas.

> 'New nurse managers are forced to wrestle with what seems to be a competition between individual patient care and organisational needs.'

Familiar situations from a new perspective

New nurse managers must look at familiar situations from a new perspective. They must adapt to:
- looking at matters 'from the inside looking out'; and
- coming to terms with an extended working environment.
  Both of these are discussed in this section of the text.

An extended working environment

To integrate clinical routines with organisational systems, the new nurse manager requires a change of 'mind-set'—thinking in a different way. It involves a change from a focus on the patient to a more general consideration of the overall organisational situation. Quality patient care remains the priority for nurse managers, but they also need to understand the way in which systems operate if they are to work within financial limits and to liaise effectively between their unit and the organisation.

> ' . . . a change from a focus on the patient to a more general consideration of the overall organisational situation.'

It is a major step to move from a patient-focused 'micro-perspective' to a 'macro-perspective' that contextualises the patient within the whole organisation. It requires an understanding of competing priorities, as well as an appreciation of the mechanics of systems—and many new nurse managers can initially feel overwhelmed. Assimilation of facts while positioning people and processes requires high-order thinking.

Situations not previously encountered or anticipated

Survival

Many organisations provide an orientation program for new nurse managers. This is a formal or informal program that focuses on specific workplace practices, procedures, and systems to assist a new nurse manager in assimilating essential information. A new nurse manager is often assigned to an experienced manager who acts as a mentor to answer specific queries and clarify issues.

Individuals who are promoted within an organisation commonly assume that they already have the requisite knowledge about the organisation. During orientation, they might therefore pay less attention to information that appears to be superficially familiar. To avoid such loss of interest, an effective and well-focused orientation program integrates appropriate role-specific material together with important current organisational information. Because the responsibilities of nurse managers extend to the wider organisation, less-familiar areas of the organisation are discussed from a manager's perspective—in addition to more familiar material about an individual practice area.

There are circumstances when a unit manager routinely deputises for a more senior manager. A relatively new nurse manager can be the senior nurse on duty during evenings, weekends, or public holidays—especially in smaller facilities. Frequently nurse managers coordinate hospitals and other health services outside the regular hours worked by administrative and departmental staff. Many hospitals do not have a resident doctor. The nurse manager in charge is often responsible for calling-in medical and other professional colleagues. There are usually organisational policies and procedures that address when and how this happens.

'If a new nurse manager proactively accesses key resources, this can minimise future confusion and save time.'

If an orientation program is not available, a new nurse manager will still need to acquire the information.

If a new nurse manager proactively accesses key resources, this can minimise future confusion and save time. In some facilities, all the necessary information is available, but its location is a mystery. It is important to know what key information should be asked for, and who to ask for it. Essential information includes:

▶ details about call systems;
▶ being able to access patient files;
▶ calling in staff to cover for sickness;
▶ accessing pharmacy, the operating theatre, and other departments; and
▶ dealing with a range of emergencies outside general business hours.

New situations

New nurse managers must cope with new situations not previously experienced. These include:

- 'survival' skills—learning about such matters as: (i) details about call systems; (ii) being able to access patient files; (iii) calling in staff to cover for sickness; (iv) accessing pharmacy, the operating theatre, and other departments; and (v) dealing with a range of emergencies outside general business hours.
- new working hours; and
- extended responsibilities—including after-hours availability.

Each of these is discussed in this section of the text.

Working hours

The shift times that nurse managers work might be determined by the organisation. Alternatively, there can be some flexibility if an appropriate rationale can be provided. Changes to work routines can result in changes to personal routines. Usually this affects others. Clear information on new working hours and planning ahead for the change can help to minimise confusion and stress.

Extended responsibilities

At the end of a shift, a clinical nurse usually hands over clinical responsibilities directly to another clinical colleague. In a similar way, ongoing management responsibilities are handed over. However, each nurse manager has a specific role that is not wholly duplicated by others. Sometimes specific after-hours queries need to be answered and, if available, the relevant nurse manager will be contacted. Leaving a contact number with clinical colleagues is not essential, but can be expedient.

In an emergency situation, a nurse manager might need to return to the workplace. This should be an unusual occurrence. With appropriate prospective planning, the nurse manager can often avoid having to be called back.

Occasionally, if there has been an unexpected event in the workplace (such as a fire or the unexpected death of a patient), a staff member might contact the off-duty nurse manager of the ward or unit. This is often merely a courtesy call to inform the manager what has happened. Other calls might be from colleagues seeking support or guidance at crucial times. There are no universally applicable rules about such situations—but many employers have established protocols. Understanding the capacity and strengths of colleagues can be helpful when making on-the-spot decisions of how to proceed.

Situations that other nurse managers deal with effectively

Being different

It is possible for different managers to achieve different outcomes from comparable situations—with neither doing anything inappropriate or incorrect. The knowledge, experience, and personal qualities of each individual influence thinking, feelings, and actions. Selecting and acknowledging the individual strengths of other managers is a way of using their experiences to advance personal skills.

> 'Selecting and acknowledging the individual strengths of other managers is a way of using their experiences to advance personal skills.'

Recording personal experiences in a journal, and reflecting on them, allows for comparisons over time. Debriefing with other managers, especially after stressful events, can be therapeutic as well as being a learning experience. Eventually a pattern of routines becomes clear, along with the occurrence of infrequent challenging events. Even within the pattern, the uniqueness of each experience is highlighted, as is the individuality of response required for each situation.

Talking things through with colleagues

Discussions with colleagues are frequently used by nurses for airing issues of concern and seeking information. In hospitals, nursing schools, and colleges, groups of nurses discuss their experiences and learn from each other. Continuing this practice into a career as a nurse manager is important. Peer support and the pooling of experiences can bring perspective to a novel situation. Management practice can be validated by realising that colleagues have worked through similar circumstances—both unpleasant and enjoyable. Differences in approach can often be seen as being due to the personalities involved, rather than the issues. Discussing coping strategies with colleagues can be invaluable.

Situations that other nurse managers cope with

New nurse managers must cope with situations that other nurse managers deal with effectively—but which a new manager finds challenging in the unaccustomed role. Such situations require:
- acceptance that everyone is different;
- talking things through with colleagues;
- an effective system of workplace supervision; and
- an effective mentoring system.
Each of these is discussed in this section of the text.

If real benefit is to be gained from such a discussion group, any censure should be minimal and support should be maximised. If one person brings a specific personal issue into a general discussion, interest often wanes, and the group is likely to break up.

Workplace supervision

Qualified nurses employed by healthcare organisations become part of that organisation's hierarchical structure, and each nurse usually has an identified supervisor or manager. Nurse managers are not only expected to supervise junior staff, but also usually have an immediate supervisor themselves.

The nature of the relationships between nurses and their immediate supervisors depends on the specific personalities involved. The personality of the supervisor, together with that person's skill and confidence in the role, determine the effectiveness of the supervision. At one end of the spectrum, supportive supervisors use quality nursing practice to guide a nurse's ongoing development. In contrast, less-effective supervisors criticise practice shortcomings and provide only grudging praise.

Depending on the nature of the relationship and the effectiveness of the supervision, junior nurses are more or less likely to consult with their supervisors when professional and personal difficulties arise.

If junior staff members present information that potentially compromises the organisation, a supervisor is in a difficult position. If a nurse discusses a legal or ethical issue with a supervisor, it might not be possible for the nurse manager to maintain the degree of confidentiality that the junior nurse anticipated. Appropriate training and experience can improve a nurse manager's confidence and effectiveness in handling these sorts of difficult issues—and others that arise in a supervisory role.

Mentoring

As in all other areas of nursing, it is important that a new nurse manager seeks out a mentor—a trusted professional friend. Many clinical nurses discuss professional issues with peers and derive support from such discussion. For nurse managers, former peers are seldom the most appropriate colleagues to respond to managerial dilemmas and issues.

'As in all other areas of nursing, it is important that a new nurse manager seeks out a mentor—a trusted professional friend.'

A mentor might be a colleague within the same organisation or might be a professional colleague who works elsewhere. Developing a trusting relationship with a colleague to talk about issues—not personalities—can be a great help, especially to a new nurse manager. It is wise to organise a definite schedule of meetings for discussion—and adherence to the agreed frequency, location, and duration of mentorship meetings reinforces their importance.

Ideally, management mentors have some training, but often circumstances dictate who is available. Talking to a colleague personally might be more appropriate than communicating by letter or email, but every situation is different. Sometimes email communications or letter-writing are more appropriate. However, committing some issues 'to paper' is not always ideal.

Conclusion

It is wise to prepare to become a nurse manager before actually achieving promotion to the position. Growth into a managerial role can be exciting; however, it can also change relationships within the workplace.

Every new nurse manager's response to the situations that he or she encounters will be based on personal knowledge and personal growth. By maintaining an effective dialogue with colleagues, together with careful planning, many of the otherwise new and unexpected circumstances in a nurse manager's day will be more challenging than stressful.

Chapter 3
Managing Ethically

Laurie Hardingham

Introduction

There are many issues in contemporary nursing that involve far-reaching ethical issues—such as informed consent, substitute decision-making, effective use of healthcare resources, moral distress of staff, and conflict between staff and family. This chapter examines some common ethical issues that nursing managers face, the notion of a moral community, and ways to combat moral distress among staff.

The nature of ethical issues

Ethical issues arise when actions are looked at from the perspective of what is 'good' and 'right'—with a view to ascertaining what should be done in specific situations. Ethical issues differ from legal issues, practical issues, medical issues, and other nursing issues in that they have to do with how others are treated, what values and beliefs are held by the people in the situations, and what principles (or rules of conduct) influence professional and personal life.

Bioethics is a relatively new field. It can be defined (Secker 2002) as involving critical reflection on the moral/ethical problems faced in healthcare settings with a view to:

▶ deciding *what* should be done (what actions are morally right or acceptable);

▶ explaining *why* it should be done (justifying the decision in moral terms); and

▶ describing *how* it should be done (the method or manner of response).

Those who work in clinical ethics do not view themselves as being the *experts* on moral issues. Rather, their role is to act as a resource to help healthcare communities build their capacities to deal with the ethical issues that are faced on a daily basis. Healthcare providers make ethical decisions throughout the day—although frequently they do not recognise the ethical components of decision-making. Deciding what to do in response to ethical questions involves many people, and ethics is an essential part of decision-making in every aspect of health care. Strengthening the capacity of healthcare teams to recognise the ethical dimensions of care and to make sound ethical decisions are important components of a nurse manager's responsibility.

> 'Ethics is an essential part of decision-making in every aspect of health care.'

Bioethics

Bioethics involves:
- deciding *what* should be done (what actions are morally right or acceptable);
- explaining *why* it should be done (justifying the decision in moral terms); and
- describing *how* it should be done (the method or manner of response).

Secker (2002)

The basis of ethical practice is an understanding that human beings are essentially *interrelated*, and that the ability to act with moral integrity (both personally and professionally) is therefore *relational* in nature. This understanding of integrity assists in appreciating what it means to act ethically in health care, and assists nurse managers in nurturing and facilitating moral reflection and action among their staff members.

Ethical, practical, legal, and administrative problems

Difficult ethical problems in health care are often framed as being either practical problems or moral dilemmas (Webster & Baylis 2001).

Practical problems include legal and administrative problems. These might include, for example, finding enough nurses to fill vacant positions, or meeting legal obligations in providing a proper standard of nursing care.

Moral dilemmas arise when there are obligations to pursue two (or more) conflicting courses of action—with no obvious reason for preferring one or other course of action. Moral dilemmas also arise when there is evidence to suggest that a particular course of action is morally right, but other evidence to suggest that it is morally wrong—with the evidence for each position being inconclusive. For example, a moral dilemma might arise between a nurse's commitment to respect a patient's autonomy and the nurse's commitment to promote that patient's best interests. This might arise if the patient's wishes conflict with what the nurse believes to be in the patient's best interests.

Ethical issues and *legal issues* are closely linked, and following the law is usually ethical. However, following the law can sometimes lead to reflection on whether it is the *right* thing to do. For example, a nurse might be reluctant to report suspected child abuse to the authorities—which, in many jurisdictions, is required by law—because he or she might lose the trust of the family and discourage family members from seeking medical help for their children in the future. The nurse's values might suggest that the ethical thing to do would be to work closely with family members to determine whether there is actual abuse, and to assist them in obtaining the resources they need to resolve their problems.

However, *practical problems* and *moral dilemmas* do not fully describe what nurses experience as 'ethical' in their practice. There are other kinds of experiences that nurses experience as 'ethical'. These can be described as:

▶ moral uncertainty;
▶ moral distress; and
▶ moral residue.

Moral uncertainty occurs when ' . . . one is unsure what moral principles or values apply, or even what the moral problem is' (Jameton 1984, p. 6). Nurses most often express this as a 'hunch'—a feeling that something is 'not quite right'. When moral uncertainty is present, sometimes all that is required is more information

'Nurses often express this as a "hunch"—a feeling that something is "not quite right".'

to bring clarity to a situation to allow for a successful resolution. If so, it might be determined that the issue is not an ethical one, but one in which *administrative change* is needed (such as recruiting more staff).

Moral uncertainty, moral distress, and moral residue

Moral uncertainty

Moral uncertainty occurs when a nurse is unsure what moral principles or values apply, or even what the moral problem is. Nurses most often express this as a 'hunch'—a feeling that something is 'not quite right'.

Moral distress

Moral distress arises when there is an inconsistency between a nurse's beliefs and actions. This is usually because the nurse knows the right thing to do, but institutional constraints make it nearly impossible to pursue the right course of action. This includes situations in which a nurse fails to do the right thing (or fails to do it to his or her satisfaction).

Moral residue

Moral residue is that which nurses carry with them from the times in their lives when (in the face of moral distress) they have seriously compromised themselves or allowed themselves to be compromised.

Moral distress arises when there is an inconsistency between one's beliefs and one's actions. For Jameton (1984, p. 6), this is usually because ' . . . one knows the right thing to do, but institutional constraints make it nearly impossible to pursue the right course of action'. Webster and Baylis (2000) broadened this definition to include situations in which one fails to do the right thing (or fails to do it to one's satisfaction) for one or more of the following reasons: (i) an error of judgment; (ii) a personal failing (such as a weakness in one's character); or (iii) other circumstances that are truly beyond one's control. In such situations, people are unable to do the right thing.

When moral distress leads to compromised integrity, Webster and Baylis (2000, p. 218) proposed the notion of *moral residue*—'that which each of us carries with us from those times in our lives when in the face of moral distress we have seriously compromised ourselves or allowed ourselves to be compromised'. Moral residue can be profound and lasting, and is usually very painful. It is an '. . . experience of compromised integrity that involves the setting aside or violation of deeply held (and

> 'Moral residue can be profound and lasting, and is usually very painful.'

publicly professed) beliefs, values, and principles [that] can sear the heart (Webster & Baylis 2000, p. 223).

Many nurses will have experienced ethical difficulties that led to moral residue for them. For example, nurses can be distressed if they feel that the nursing care they are asked to give is against their patient's wishes, or if they feel that they are performing therapeutic interventions that patients do not want. Nurses can find themselves going home at the end of their shift and feeling upset and helpless about the care that they have provided to some of their patients. They find themselves thinking about these patients frequently, and linking them to past events—for example, patients who continued to be treated intensively against their will, and who subsequently died months later in great pain. The new case can thus recall memories of previous patients, and many nurses relive the stress they felt at that time.

Moral integrity

The word 'integrity' is derived from the Latin *integer* (meaning 'whole'). Having integrity means that a person is a 'whole person'. Moral integrity, personal or professional, is thus about 'wholeness' in the relationship between that person's actions and the person's values and our beliefs. Moral integrity is about a certain 'whole' conception that the person has of himself or herself.

> 'Moral integrity is about "wholeness" in the relationship between a person's actions and that person's values and our beliefs.'

There are three aspects to moral integrity (May 1996):

▶ critical thinking;
▶ coherence of value orientation; and
▶ a disposition or commitment to act in a principled way.

The first aspect, *critical thinking*, relates to the definition of bioethics given above. Being able to explain the 'what', 'why', and 'how' of one's ethical decisions requires that nurses reflect on (and be able to articulate to others) the process of their decision-making regarding the right thing to do. This takes skill, knowledge, and practice.

The second aspect, *coherence*, means that a person with integrity can be relied upon to act in a way that is responsive to a well-thought-out view of the relation between his or her beliefs and actions. Moral integrity should not be seen as holding steadfastly to a code of conduct that others have provided—even if the person approves of this code. Rather, moral integrity should be viewed as maturing by reflection on many different values—thus providing a critical coherence to the experience that one has (May 1996). This means developing a critical perspective—a standpoint from which one can examine new social influences, and then endorse or reject them. Individuals need to be thoughtful and reflective as they develop values and accept standards regarding how to live their lives. Nurses should also participate in thoughtful conversations about the values and theories that guide nursing actions and attitudes—something that cannot be done in isolation. For nurses, this process must begin in their nursing education, continue with their socialisation into the profession, and then become an inherent part of their nursing practice. Supporting this process is a key element of ethical management.

> 'Developing a critical perspective—a standpoint from which one can examine new social influences, and then endorse or reject them.'

Moral integrity

There are three aspects to moral integrity:
- critical thinking;
- coherence of value orientation; and
- a disposition or commitment to act in a principled way.
  Each of these is discussed in this section of the text.

The third aspect, the *commitment to act in a principled way*, must also be supported by the nurse manager. When nurses are prevented from actions that match their principles, the moral distress that arises can affect the morale of the healthcare community and the kind of care that patients are given.

The challenges to integrity in health care are not merely theoretical (Chambliss 1996). Moral and ethical challenges in nursing are systemic features of contemporary hospitals, and these features are a normal part of hospital operations—rather than external or accidental (Chambliss 1996). An organisation's structure determines both *what* are perceived as problems and *how* those problems are managed.

> 'Moral and ethical challenges in nursing are systemic features of contemporary hospitals—rather than external or accidental.'

Two empirical observations are of interest when thinking about moral integrity (Chambliss 1996).

▶ Nursing's ethical problems are systematic. What nurses see as ethical problems arise in predictable settings, over and over again. They are not random events. As Chambliss (1996, p. 91) observed: ' . . . remove a nurse with an ethical problem from the hospital, replace her, and her replacement will encounter the same problem. The problem is not of the person but of the system.'

▶ Nurses face practical difficulties, not private dilemmas. What is involved is the practical problem of accomplishing some task over the ' . . . opposition of other people: a recalcitrant physician, a family that doesn't understand, administrators who must meet budgets' (Chambliss 1996, p. 92). Nurses know what should be done, but they just cannot do it.

These observations emphasise that ethical problems in health care are inseparable from the organisational and social settings in which they arise. One of the implications of this is that 'the assumption of relatively autonomous decision makers is simply unrealistic . . . Since the great problems of health care are structural and not the result of poor reasoning, the solutions cannot be created by increasing education, holding ethics seminars, or (alas) writing books' (Chambliss 1996, p. 183).

How graduate nurses perceive their adaptation to the 'real world' of hospital nursing is particularly illuminating of how the struggle to maintain moral integrity is a complex process that depends on the psychosocial environment of nurses (Kelly 1996). In the early years after graduation, self-doubt and confusion from intense stress can result in greater reliance on others as references for self-evaluation. Individual ethical standards are influenced by group norms, and the environment in which nurses work

> 'The practice and support of more experienced colleagues is of the utmost importance in professional values and identity.'

(as well as the practice and support of their more experienced colleagues) is of the utmost importance in the maintenance of professional values and a professional identity (Kelly 1996).

The *social climate of the hospital unit* in which nurses practise is of great significance. As students, nurses appear to internalise a sense of responsibility to uphold the standards that they have been taught, and they expect a great deal of themselves (Kelly 1996). However, they come to believe in their first years in practice that ethical compromise is unavoidable in hospital nursing. If nurses find themselves unable to conform to ward routines and to the norms of the team (or more particularly the values of the charge nurse), they are forced to move to another job or out of the profession: ' . . . maintaining professional standards in hospitals is not easy' (Kelly 1996, p. 1067).

Moral integrity does not therefore depend only on the individual living up to norms and standards. Rather, it is embedded in social practice. If morality is, indeed, rooted in collective life, a nurse's ability to have integrity ultimately rests within the kind of community of which the nurse is part. To take ethical concerns forwards in a clinical setting, the participants must build a 'moral community'—a community in which there is no gap between what participants know is the right thing to do and what they actually do.

> 'A "moral community" is a community in which there is no gap between what participants know is the right thing to do and what they actually do.'

Building moral communities

Integrity requires critical reflection with others. Unfortunately, in modern healthcare organisations professionals often do not have a safe place (or the time or inclination) to do this work of critical reflection. One of the ways of maintaining integrity is to create and strengthen a moral community in which to do this work.

A moral community is (Webster & Baylis 2000, p. 228):

> . . . a community in which there is coherence between what a healthcare organization publicly professes to be—namely, helping, healing, caring environments that embrace the virtues intrinsic to the practice of healthcare—and what employees, patients and others both witness and participate in.

Forming such a community would go a long way to reducing moral distress and moral residue on the part of all people working in it.

What would such a moral community look like? And how would a nurse manager work towards building and strengthening his or her particular community to become a moral one? This is a question with no easy answer, but the International Council of Nurses' definition of nursing might be a beginning (see Box, page 31).

Definition of nursing

Nursing encompasses autonomous and collaborative care of individuals of all ages, families, groups and communities, sick or well and in all settings. Nursing includes the promotion of health, prevention of illness, and the care of ill, disabled and dying people. Advocacy, promotion of a safe environment, research, participation in shaping health policy and in patient and health systems management, and education are also key nursing roles.

International Council of Nurses (2000)

This definition speaks of 'autonomous and collaborative care . . . advocacy, promotion of a safe environment . . . participation in shaping health policy and in patient and health systems management' as being key nursing roles. The emphasis is on *collective* action. Although autonomous care also plays a role, the definition suggests a shift in focus within nursing ethics—from the ethical obligations of the individual nurse to an approach that shifts attention to the social relations within an organisation and how institutions distribute power.

> ' . . . an approach that shifts attention to the social relations within an organisation and how institutions distribute power.'

Organisations declare what really counts by their treatment of staff, the institutional goals they set, and how they handle controversy and conflicts. Ethical analysis should be part of the administrative, policymaking, and interpersonal aspects of organisational life if it is to bridge the gap between professional values taught during the formal socialisation process and application of these values in complex clinical settings. In this way the organisation will assume some responsibility for helping those new to the organisation and for reducing moral distress (Reiser 1994).

A valuable exercise for the nurse manager would be to examine his or her organisation's mission statement (what the organisation does), vision (what the organisation will be), and values (how the organisation serves its purpose; the foundation for all decision-making). The public, patients, families, and staff are told that the organisation will live up to these statements.

One of the first questions to ask is whether there is coherence between these statements and the actions that people in the community live and see every day. This should be asked of everyone working within the organisation in a way that facilitates reflection and discussion, and the questioner must listen to what is said. Feelings must be sought about the mission and values, and about working in the organisation. Unless feelings are dealt with, solutions cannot be suggested. In health care, feelings are never far from the surface and, if not articulated, can lead to conflict. This is because most situations in health care involve difficult circumstances to deal with, and many value-based decisions have to be made.

There are also many different professional backgrounds, status, and power differences, and various roles and responsibilities of team members. The only way to engage *all* members of the healthcare team in the resolution of a problem might involve allowing all of them to express their feelings to each other—so that everyone can understand the deep feelings that the situation has engendered. Without this understanding, it is very difficult to come up with a process to resolve the problem. In many cases, when feelings are articulated and dealt with, the team members will have the energy to find constructive solutions.

Opening up the 'moral space' for such discussions to take place is not an easy task—but one that is worth pursuing. A set of useful principles known as the 'Tavistock Principles' has been developed for all of those involved in health care—rather than the more common principles that have been developed for only one discipline, such as nursing. Among these principles (see Box, below) are cooperation, improvement, and openness. These three principles all require that healthcare staff be open to learning, change, and working together—and sharing ideas, values, and beliefs with honesty and openness.

The Tavistock Principles

Rights—people have a right to health and health care.

Balance—care of individual patients is central, but the health of populations is also our concern.

Comprehensiveness—in addition to treating illness, we have an obligation to ease suffering, minimise disability, prevent disease, and promote health.

Cooperation—health care succeeds only if we cooperate with those we serve, each other, and those in other sectors.

Improvement—improving health care is a serious and continuing responsibility.

Safety—do no harm.

Openness—being open, honest, and trustworthy is vital in health care.

Berwick et al. (2001, p. 616)

Resource allocation

Decisions on resource allocation are increasingly becoming a topic of concern for nurse managers and all those who work in health care. It is a common misperception that such decisions are made only at the administrative level. These decisions are also made every day by many people who work in the frontlines of health care. Examples include deciding how to divide one's time among patients, or deciding whether to use a more expensive or less expensive kind of wound dressing. These decisions have important consequences for individuals, organisations, and societies.

'Resource-allocation decisions are made every day by many people who work in the frontlines of health care.'

There are three levels of decision-making in resource allocation.

▶ *Micro-allocation decisions* take place at the individual level, and concern the distribution of resources such as treatments, drugs, or procedures to individuals in need. At this level individual practitioners make decisions every day about what individual patients need and what they will receive. If resources could be distributed solely according to need, decisions made at this level would be easy. However, many constraints are placed on decision-making—including scarcity of beds, materials, drugs, and human resources.

▶ *Meso-allocation decisions* are those made at an institutional or community level. Decisions such as which programs will be funded in a community and how the available resources will be divided within a region are examples of meso-allocation.

▶ *Macro-allocation decisions* are those related to broader public policy decisions—such as how much money a government will allocate to health care and which priorities it will set for use of that money. An example is whether to prioritise prevention of illness over cure of illness.

An important concept when looking at decision-making levels is that the decisions made at each level will affect the decisions that can be made at other levels. For example, admitting a patient to an intensive care unit (ICU) bed will mean that that bed will not be available for other patients. Moreover, it might require the institution to consider increasing the number of ICU beds. Decisions about decreasing funding to public health can make it difficult for providers to provide preventive health care (such as immunisation) to the individuals for whom they are responsible.

Decisions on resource allocation also require an environment in which people who work at the different levels can engage in open dialogue and share values—

an important component of a moral community (CNA 2000). It is also necessary to have a commitment to a principle-based approach to decision-making that will assist people to make good decisions.

Resources for nurse managers in ethical decision-making

Principles for decision-making

The Tavistock Principles (see page 32) are relatively new principles that attempt to provide decision-making guidance for all those involved in health care. In the relatively short history of bioethics, four principles have predominated (Beauchamp & Childress 2001):

▶ *beneficence*: having to do with doing good, providing benefits, and balancing benefits against risks and costs;

▶ *non-malfeasance*: avoiding causing harm;

▶ *justice*: distributing benefits, risks, and costs fairly; and

▶ *respect for autonomy*: respecting the decision-making of autonomous persons.

Resources for ethical decision-making

The following resources for nurse managers in ethical decision-making are discussed in this section of the text:

• principles for decision-making;
• professional associations;
• codes of ethics;
• past issues and cases;
• bioethicists and healthcare ethics centres;
• religious and chaplaincy services;
• educational institutions and departments;
• core organisational values and policies; and
• the law.

Professional associations

Most countries have a nursing professional association—the responsibility of which is to regulate nursing care to protect the public. In addition, the International Council of Nurses is an organisation with a mission to ' . . . represent nursing worldwide, advancing the profession and influencing health policy' (ICN 2003). The *ICN Code for Nurses* provides a 'foundation for ethical nursing practice throughout the world' (ICN 2003).

Many professional associations offer models, frameworks, or guidelines for ethical decision-making, and make them available on their websites.

Codes of ethics

National and international nursing associations have written codes of ethics—which are meant to provide a framework for decision-making for nurses in practice, management, research, and education. Although such codes are necessarily vague and general, they can provide a basis for reflection, discussion, and debate when ethical issues come up.

Past issues and cases

Difficult ethical dilemmas and issues that have occurred in an organisation make excellent case studies of how to improve ethical decision-making in the future. Case studies can assist healthcare providers to devise processes to decrease the possibility of such problems recurring. For problems that cannot be prevented, managers and staff can be educated on how the problems can be better resolved.

Bioethicists and healthcare ethics centres

Although many healthcare organisations around the world do not have access to the services of a bioethicist or an ethics centre, the study of bioethics is an emerging field and is recognised internationally as a resource to assist healthcare providers in addressing the many value-laden issues that occur in health care. There is a large amount of written material and other resources available—both in print and on the Internet. In addition, there are many individuals and organisations who will consult with those in need of such services. Many ethics centres have decision-making models to help people in making difficult decisions.

Religious and chaplaincy services

Religious leaders and spiritual-care providers have a tradition of studying ethical theory, asking ethical questions, and of helping people work through difficult and sensitive issues.

Educational institutions and departments

Universities, colleges, business schools, nursing schools, and hospital education departments can offer many resources to nurse managers on ethics, moral theory, and good decision-making models.

Core organisational values and policies

As noted above (page 31), core organisational values and mission statements can provide a guide to decision-making—particularly if they have been well thought-out and if they provide direction that can actually be put into practice. An organisation's policies and procedures manual can also be helpful; if it is not, it can become the basis of a discussion on what needs to be changed.

The law

The *law* has been listed last—because the law can be viewed as 'minimal ethics'. In other words, the law is more likely to tell a person what he or she should *not* do; it less likely to provide answers as to what that person *should* do. The law is therefore not always helpful for ethical questions, and nor does it necessarily address *all* questions. However, if the law does give guidance in a situation, it is a good place to start when trying to make a decision.

Conclusion

There are no easy answers when ethical issues arise in health care, and nurse managers must do the work of ethical analysis, reflection, and exploration of options if they are to come up with good ethical resolutions to ethical problems.

One of the most important ways of promoting good ethical practice is to create an environment in which everyone can participate in the articulation of values and in making decisions on the process of putting those values into practice. In such an environment, anyone who is unsure whether the right thing is being done can raise a 'red flag'.

Helping to create a moral community in which people can do this, and in which there is coherence between what an organisation professes to do and what it is actually doing in practice, is one of the most important ethical obligations of a nurse manager.

> 'Helping to create a moral community . . . is one of the most important ethical obligations of a nurse manager.'

Chapter 4

Leading, Motivating, and Enthusing

Mike Musker

Introduction

A new nurse manager is often plunged into the unfamiliar role of leading a group of people while being simultaneously expected to know all relevant policies and procedures, observe occupational health-and-safety rules, and be aware of legal responsibilities. In addition to all of these responsibilities, the new nurse manager has to face the complex task of managing people. In many cases, the only training that new nurse managers receive is 'on-the-job' experience. Learning in these circumstances becomes a matter of learning through mistakes—which often leads to anxiety and stress.

Against this background, learning to lead can be a daunting prospect for the new nurse manager. However, learning how to lead is, in essence, no different from learning the other skills that form part of the nurse manager's repertoire.

Theories of leadership

Over the years, several theories of leadership have emerged. These can be summarised as follows:

▶ *trait theory*: according to which leaders possess specific inherent qualities and behaviours; usually associated with a long list of positive attributes;

▶ *'great man' theory*: according to which leadership is an inherited condition possessed by great leaders; leaders are thus born not made;

▶ *situational theory*: according to which every situation requires a specific type of leadership to fit the context and environment; the leader adapts his or her style according to the situation and the players involved (Hersey & Blanchard 1993);

▶ *contingency theory*: according to which there is an interaction among leader–follower relationships, the structure of the task, and positional power; leaders who are fixed in their style work better with some team members than others (Fiedler & Chemers 1974); and

▶ *path–goal leadership*: according to which leadership clarifies the path and removes obstacles in achieving objectives or goals; the leader analyses the team member's expectations of the task and identifies valued rewards (House 1971).

From these models, two major leadership styles have emerged:

▶ transactional leadership; and

▶ transformational leadership.

Transactional leadership is a functional approach that reviews the needs of the group, the task, and the individual. This model focuses on the *function* of leadership in achieving a task, taking into account the needs of individuals and the needs of the group (Adair 1983). The components of this model include (Henderson, Phillips & Lewis 2000):

▶ *planning*: drawing together all the information required;

▶ *initiating*: getting together with the team and sharing the task;

▶ *controlling*: measuring what is happening and where the team is up to; and

▶ *supporting*: providing the motivation where required.

Transformational leadership is a humanistic approach that involves a combination of charisma, belief, style, and vision. This focuses on the relationship of the leader with team members—especially the leader's ability to provide inspiration. Transformational leadership is the preferred style in the caring professions—in which the emphasis is on relationships with people. In this regard, the following aspects of transformational leadership are especially significant:

Two major types of leadership

Two major leadership styles are discussed in this section of the text:
- transactional leadership; and
- transformational leadership.

Transactional leadership

This model focuses on *achieving a task*, taking into account the needs of individuals and the needs of the group.

Transformational leadership

This model focuses on the *relationship of the leader with team members*—especially the leader's ability to provide inspiration. This is the preferred style in the caring professions.

- creating and expressing an exciting vision for a team;
- motivating and enthusing people to embrace this vision;
- using charisma, being respected, and having integrity;
- showing creativity, ingenuity, and innovation;
- sharing power and empowering others;
- working across boundaries and disciplines;
- bringing vitality, belief, and inspiration;
- empowering, enabling, and involving the team;
- being confident, self-assured, and courageous;
- showing concern for people in terms of their personal and professional needs;
- having an ability to tap into individual resources;
- being able to rise above and review situations (the so-called 'helicopter trait');
- exuding professionalism (while remaining approachable); and
- thriving in a crisis and finding solutions.

These traits are not necessarily innate, and people can develop them through lifelong learning. Employers have a responsibility to their employees to provide for their personal development, and most organisations now offer opportunities to attend leadership courses. Leadership courses should be available to future managers as well as current managers (Fister-Gale 2002), and everyone in

'Everyone in an organisation should be given opportunities to lead, regardless of position and status.'

an organisation should be given opportunities to lead, regardless of position and status.

Strategies of transformational leadership

The characteristics of transformational leadership described above lend themselves to certain strategies of leadership. For the nurse manager, the following strategies are especially useful:

▶ sharing a vision;

▶ avoiding the quest for popularity; and

▶ being aware of power.

Each of these is discussed below.

Sharing a vision

Nurse managers should create a vision that is shared by the team. To achieve this, managers need the ability to tap into the imagination of team members and produce a vision in which they all believe—not something that senior managers want to hear.

A transformational leader must be committed to the values and beliefs of the vision, and must be consistent in demonstrating this commitment. Such a manager will enlighten, inspire, and become a role model for others (Hall 2002). Team members need a leader with whom they feel confident and who shows confidence in them (Hersey & Blanchard 1993).

Three strategies of transformational leadership

Three major strategies of transformational leadership are discussed in this section of the text:

- sharing a vision;
- avoiding the quest for popularity; and
- being aware of power.

Avoiding the quest for popularity

People sometimes require direction to complete unpopular tasks. If someone has to be asked to complete a difficult chore or if it is necessary to deal with unsatisfactory performance, this should not be put off. The manager should be direct, open, and honest, rather than procrastinate and worry about how the issue will be broached. People expect their superiors to express their displeasure when necessary—as long as this is done professionally and courteously.

Being aware of power

Exercising responsibility invariably involves exercising power, and knowing how to use power appropriately is an ongoing challenge for nurse managers. It is helpful to characterise power in the following terms:

▶ legitimate (or positional) power;
▶ reward (or resource) power;
▶ referent (or personal) power;
▶ expert power;
▶ negative power; and
▶ coercive power.

Each of these is discussed below.

Legitimate (or positional) power

Legitimate (or *positional*) *power* is the power given through status and position within an organisation. There should be little need for a transformational manager to use this type of power; however, at times, this can become necessary (Kosinska & Niebroj 2003).

Reward (or resource) power

With positional power usually comes control of resources—such as access to courses. This is known as *reward* (or *resource*) *power*.

The fact that a nurse manager has the power to authorise the use of resources can induce those who want that resource to engage in ingratiating behaviour, or to express disappointment or resentment if they do not receive it. It is essential that the nurse manager initiates an authorisation system that is transparent and equitable.

Five forms of power

Five forms of power are discussed in this section of the text:

• legitimate (or positional) power;
• reward (or resource) power;
• referent (or personal) power;
• expert power;
• negative power; and
• coercive power.

Referent (or personal) power

Referent (or *personal*) *power* must be earned through respect for the way in which situations are managed. This sort of power is obtained through reputation and experience.

Natural 'charisma' is a trait that is often associated with this form of power, but personal power can be obtained over time. New managers should be patient in their attempts to achieve respect. It can take several years to achieve. In the meantime, nurse managers have greater reliance on positional power in the early part of their careers.

> 'New managers should be patient in their attempts to achieve respect. It can take several years to achieve.'

Expert power

Expert power is exercised through having the appropriate experience, knowledge, and skills for the leadership role. Staff members often look to their leader for guidance—and expect the manager to have the answers.

The nurse manager should therefore keep up to date with the latest research and evidenced-based practice. However, it is not necessary to know everything or pretend to know everything. The nurse manager should be honest in admitting gaps in knowledge, but should ensure that access to the required information is available and facilitated.

> 'It is not necessary to know everything or pretend to know everything.'

In addition, the nurse manager should respect the expertise of others in the team, and should ensure that their knowledge is shared as a resource.

Negative power

Negative power refers to power based on a complex hierarchical chain of command in an organisation, This sort of power can actually prevent things being achieved because the complexity of the chain of command prevents the efficient utilisation of human and physical resources.

Coercive power

The term *coercive power* is used in two ways. It can refer to the power to block something because a person occupies a certain strategic position in a chain of events required for the completion of a task. It can also be used to refer to the executive power to use 'force' to stop something happening (Handy 1999).

Motivation

Motivating factors

Motivation is what makes people want to do their job. Apart from the desire to earn a living, people are motivated in their jobs by (Falcone 2002):

▶ a desire for personal development;
▶ enjoyment of a safe and pleasant environment;
▶ having opportunities for educational development;
▶ a desire for respect and recognition; and
▶ the enjoyment of working with a good leader.

Nursing is often referred to as a vocation—a 'calling' to help others. For many nurses, fulfilment of this calling is reward enough. However, in more difficult environments (for example, if nurses are threatened, abused, or even physically assaulted), the ideal can quickly wear off.

Maslow's hierarchy of needs

A useful theory on motivation for the nurse manager is that of Maslow (1970). This theory is based on a 'hierarchy of needs'. According to Maslow, the primary human needs are physiological (including hunger, thirst, and bodily comfort). The need for safety and security forms the next level in the hierarchy before 'higher needs' can be considered. When safety is accomplished, relationships with other people are on the next hierarchical level, and Maslow argues that it is a natural desire for a person to seek a sense of 'belonging' to a team or group. The higher levels of need relate to self-esteem and what Maslow refers to as 'self-actualisation'—a desire to reach full potential.

In the nursing workplace, these higher needs might involve being competent (or excellent) in a job, achieving high academic standards, or reaching a certain positional status. According to Maslow's model, nurses have a natural desire to be fulfilled by their roles. Work involves a significant proportion of a person's life, and organisations should provide a supportive environment in which needs can be fulfilled.

McGregor's 'X–Y theory'

Another useful model of motivation for the nurse manager is McGregor's (1960) 'X–Y theory'. This takes a dichotomous approach in which people are viewed in one of two ways. The manager might see people as being 'X people' or 'Y people'.

▶ 'X people' are people who are perceived as being indolent and resistant to change;

▶ 'Y people' are people who are perceived as wanting to achieve personal fulfilment through being productive at work.

If a manager views people as being 'Y' people, the manager is more likely to attempt to provide them with the conditions they require in which to thrive. In contrast, a manager who adopts the 'X' perspective of people will be more likely to focus on ensuring the completion of given tasks within given timeframes. According to the theory, the way in which people are viewed by the manager determines the whole focus of that person's management style.

'The way in which people are viewed by the manager determines the whole focus of that person's management style.'

Two theories of motivation

Two theories of motivation are discussed in this section of the text:
• Maslow's hierarchy of needs; and
• McGregor's 'X–Y theory'.

Mentorship and clinical supervision

Staff members look to the manager as a model for personal development. The skills portrayed by the manager are likely to be the skills that staff members want to emulate. The nurse manager should therefore be a role model of professionalism and consistency, and should always be aware that his or her words and actions are helping to shape the views of aspiring staff. The nurse manager should therefore:

▶ spend time with staff members who have potential to develop into managers;

▶ provide coaching by talking through scenarios and allowing staff members to offer solutions;

▶ work through some experiences by telling stories and anecdotes (Trofino 2000);

▶ refer problems back to staff members and encourage *them* to find a solution, rather than accepting the burden of responsibility for something that can be managed at the subordinate level; and

▶ encourage staff members to think laterally and create unconventional solutions to problems.

The nurse manager's image as a leader can have a significant effect on others. Such matters as the manager's dress and appearance, the manager's methods of dealing with people in difficult circumstances, and the manager's overall professional consistency are all important in presenting an effective image as a role model.

The art of delegation

When a manager is first given the role of being in charge of a team, he or she often finds it difficult to delegate tasks. The manager can end up running around doing everything (and becoming exhausted) while other staff members are looking for things to do.

A new manager often does not realise that giving a team member responsibility for a task can actually be rewarding for both the manager and the staff member. Sharing work is an important aspect of a team approach. It shows respect for the staff member by recognising that he or she is able to complete a task, and it provides that person with opportunities for reward.

> 'Giving a team member responsibility for a task can be rewarding for both the manager and the staff member.'

However, at the other extreme, a new team leader must not exploit others by taking every opportunity to get others to do things for the manager. An effective leader has a good knowledge of the work that he or she is delegating, and should take the opportunity, whenever possible, to demonstrate his or her own capabilities.

The way in which people are asked to do things can have a significant effect on when it is done and how well it is done. If people are treated with courtesy and respect, and with due regard for their capacities and expertise, the results are more likely to be positive.

If there are problems in getting a staff member to do a task (despite the manager's best efforts to delegate effectively), line managers should be informed of what is going on. If possible, new nurse managers should make use of manager colleagues to provide a healthy level of support.

Effective leadership

Four strategies that the nurse manager can employ in providing effective leadership for a nursing team are:

- meeting regularly and frequently with staff;
- being a good listener;
- giving praise and being aware of personal fears; and
- shadowing and keeping in practice.

Each of these is discussed below.

Meeting regularly and frequently with staff

Formal meetings with staff members as a group should be held on a regular and frequent basis either weekly or fortnightly. Such meetings can avoid or resolve work-related issues by allowing time for discussion of controversial items on the team's agenda. The meetings are also an opportunity to provide organisational policies, procedures, and other relevant information from meetings of senior management. All queries raised at the meetings should be followed through, and outcomes should be shared at the next meeting.

In addition to such formal meetings, 'management by walking about' ensures that the manager is 'visible' to staff members and that the manager is aware of what is happening in his or her area of responsibility. This is especially important if the manager has responsibility for more than one area.

The manager should adopt an 'open-door policy' that allows staff members to call in and discuss issues. Such informality provides opportunities for staff members to discuss personal issues and experiences that are causing them concern. In such a setting, staff members also often provide advice about staff dynamics within an area.

A line management structure that allows good communication should be used. Having a number of avenues for contact helps to prevent problems arising.

Four strategies of effective leadership

Four strategies of effective leadership are discussed in this section of the text:

- meeting regularly and frequently with staff;
- being a good listener;
- giving praise and being aware of personal fears; and
- shadowing and keeping in practice.

Being a good listener

When meeting with staff members the manager should be aware of the 'balance' of the conversation. The aim should be a conversation in which the staff member contributes about 70% of the input and the manager contributes about 30% (Wright 1993).

The nurse manager should listen actively to what is said, and should encourage the generation of new ideas. This ensures that staff members have a sense of 'ownership' of ideas—thus increasing motivation and interest.

Consultation with staff will help the manager to gain a different perspective on issues and obtain insight into staff members' experiences of the work situation (Neisloss 2002).

Giving praise and being aware of personal fears

Staff members require reassurance that they are doing well and that there are no plans to move them to another area. Managers should provide reward and recognition to originators of work by ensuring that names appear, as appropriate, on relevant documentation (such as business proposals and memoranda) (Thyer 2003). In providing recognition and encouraging motivation of the individuals concerned, the manager also gains in personal credibility.

Encouragement and motivation are also enhanced by giving each staff member a special area of responsibility, thus providing the person with an opportunity to thrive.

Shadowing and keeping in practice

Knowing the 'ins and outs' of every job is not easy in the increasingly complex world of the nurse manager. Despite this, managers are expected to know everything that is happening within their sphere of control (Tappen 2001). 'Shadowing' is a process whereby a senior person is followed around for a set period of time—usually a day. This can be done in both directions—a leader can 'shadow' a subordinate and/or a subordinate can 'shadow' a leader.

'Acting-up' opportunities and 'acting-down' opportunities complement this process. For example, a manager might take the opportunity to perform the role of a subordinate while that person is on holiday. This gives the manager a clearer idea of what others are expected to do. Moreover, demonstrating such an empathic attitude earns respect from subordinates and demonstrates a supportive approach.

Conclusion

It has been said that 'to manage is to control; to lead is to liberate' (Owen 1990). The nurse manager, as leader, needs to form relationships that are tailored to each member of the team. Developing an effective leadership style that is employee-centred aids in the creation of a visionary culture that empowers all staff members to lead themselves.

> 'To manage is to control; to lead is to liberate.'

Chapter 5

Working with Other Disciplines

Cynthia Stuhlmiller

Introduction

Delivery of health care is a collaborative effort, and each person has a valuable contribution to make. Although many important aspects of care are not specific to any particular discipline—for example, those that involve the basic principles of positive human interaction—other aspects are determined by the specific expertise and requirements of various disciplinary or occupational groups.

Because nurse managers are responsible for ensuring that efficient and effective nursing services are delivered, they must know how each person's role fits into the overall plan of care and must ensure that it is understood and valued by others, including the patient. An understanding of different disciplinary perspectives enables good organisational planning and can assist in dealing with the conflicts that inevitably emerge. This chapter provides a framework for appreciating fundamental differences among disciplines, explains why tensions and conflict occur, and outlines strategies for promoting good interprofessional relations.

Understanding occupational differences

The convergence of different occupations in accomplishing a shared goal is not unique to health care. In many work settings, various occupations hold distinctive knowledge and values that determine roles, expectations, customs, and goals. Individuals within each group have ties to their work that are formed and confirmed by socialisation and practices specific to the discipline in which they work. However, threats and challenges to expectations and goals can engender stress and conflict within and between these occupational groups.

'An important aspect of the role of the nurse manager is to coordinate various occupational groups to ensure smooth functioning and effective health care.'

Priority and decision-making are determined by the value and meaning of work and an individual's personal understanding of what is required to carry out a role efficiently (Stuhlmiller 1994, 1996).

An important aspect of the role of the nurse manager is to coordinate these various occupational groups to ensure smooth functioning and effective health care.

Models driving practice

Each discipline within the healthcare team has its own knowledge, and this drives the ways in which that discipline carries out its work. In health care, there are two basic models on which disciplines can base their practice. These are:

▶ the disease (or pathogenesis) model; and
▶ the health and wellness (or salutogenesis) model.

The disease model is the one that underpins the practice of medical doctors and the ways in which they give care and administer their management systems. Nursing practice is firmly based on the model of health and wellness. The wellness model is concerned with how people stay healthy—given their ever-present exposure to the possibility of disease and ill health (Antonovsky 1979, 1987). This model differs from the disease model in that it looks for factors that promote health (or *ease*), rather than those that cause ill health (or *dis-ease*). Each of these models of health care has its strengths and limitations. Few people would deny the importance of identifying the causes of disease and of treating that disease, but care of persons involves a broader perspective than this, and encompasses other forms of management.

One of the problems faced by nurse managers is that various disciplines in the healthcare team might tend to follow either the disease model or the health model, and might thus have different practices and goals. In a disease-dominated environment, there will be less emphasis on a patient's coping abilities, strengths, and resilience to ill health, and more emphasis on medical, surgical, and pharmaceutical interventions (Stuhlmiller 2000). However, because nurses deal with the complex interaction of lifestyle, environment, and social factors, the wellness model of healthcare delivery involves an investigation of factors beyond conventional disease-orientated therapeutic interventions.

Differing professional perspectives

Nurses straddle both of the above models of care provision. Traditionally, nurses have learnt about diseases, disorders, and the physiological and emotional changes that occur in life. This information enables nurses to understand the causation, signs and symptoms, and courses of diseases. However, the work of the nurse involves an investigation of a person's *understanding* of disease and *experience* of illness, with a view to assisting that person to feel at ease, cope, and regain health—to the extent that this is possible.

'The role of the nurse involves an investigation of a person's *understanding* of disease and *experience* of illness.'

Whatever model or approach is emphasised by various disciplines within the team, the nurse manager must be flexible and accommodating to ensure that the health of the patient remains the ultimate focus. Although there is considerable overlap among various healthcare disciplines, each will engage with people from a slightly different perspective. It is the role of the nurse manager to ensure that these differences in emphasis have positive outcomes on the person in care.

Role differences and disrespect

If managers do not take care to ensure that all disciplines work collaboratively, the work of each individual discipline can be disrupted, thus creating stress. For example, if a person's blood type is recorded inaccurately, the nurse responsible for administering the blood will undoubtedly feel resentment towards those who made the error. Professionals function best when they have a sense of control over their own practice. A loss of control creates personal discomfort that is usually manifested as anger in an attempt to regain a sense of control over what is happening. Failure to acknowledge differences in concerns and obligations among various disciplines results in further misunderstanding, stereotyping, and disrespect.

Different disciplines . . . different perspectives

A person who is to undergo coronary artery bypass surgery will receive care from people representing various disciplines in the healthcare team. Although all disciplines are interested in a comprehensive assessment of the person, each group will focus on specific data relevant to its particular concerns. For example:

- surgeons will be especially interested in the person's blood type, circulatory function, and so on;
- anaesthetists will have a particular interest in allergic reactions, smoking history, and general health;
- social workers will be especially interested in insurance cover, pensions, social service benefits, and so on;
- physiotherapists will have a particular interest in mobility and chest movement (especially postoperatively); and
- dietitians will be concerned about nutritional state and postoperative feeding requirements.

Nurses will also be interested in these data, as well as the person's ability to understand (and cope with) what is happening to him or her. The nurse will not only be monitoring physical signs and symptoms, but also assessing emotional and social needs. Even if the surgical procedure is a success, if the person conveys that he or she is depressed, health will be compromised.

In practice, this means that the nurse manager has to be aware of how the various disciplines work and the position that each occupies in the hierarchy of health care. With these different hierarchical positions come differences in power. To work effectively together, each discipline must demonstrate a willingness to listen to the perspectives of the others. Everyone, including the nurse manager, must be flexible enough to:

- instruct (and be instructed);
- advocate for (and allow advocacy);
- ask for advice (and advise);
- access information (and share it);
- make suggestions (and be open to the suggestions of others);
- listen (and be listened to); and
- negotiate (and be negotiated with).

These flexible work practices include collaborative strategic planning, working within established protocols, and networking effectively.

The nurse manager as nurse

In addition to ensuring that the nursing team collaborates with other disciplines, the nurse manager is also responsible for ensuring that the essential practice of nursing continues.

What nurses actually do can seem quite ordinary (Taylor 1994), but the work of nurses is fundamentally important to the overall facilitation of health and recovery. Because the involvement of nurses with those in their care is often more intimate and sustained than that of other disciplines, nurses are well placed to offer practical solutions that are relevant to the person's needs.

The nurse manager's role thus involves more than collaboration with other disciplines. It also involves ensuring the effective operation of the nursing team in the essential task of providing professional nursing care.

> 'The nurse manager's role involves collaboration with other disciplines *and* the effective operation of the nursing team in the essential task of providing professional nursing care.'

The future of interdisciplinary teamwork

The three 'Ps'

New ways of working in health care require that traditional professional élitism must be replaced with structures that promote collective commitment to quality care. Such interprofessional work encompasses the 'three Ps' of:

- philosophy;
- policy; and
- patient.

In working with other professionals, nurses must therefore (Kenny 2002):

- be explicit about their *philosophy* and values;
- participate in *policy* generation that promotes interprofessional cooperation; and
- engage in research and dialogue that places the *patient* at the centre of care delivery.

The members of each healthcare discipline will have a loyalty to their own profession. However, the ultimate loyalty of all must be to the *patient* and his or her care. *Philosophies* and *policies* might differ in detail, but they are all ultimately informed by the overall goal of serving the needs of the *patient*.

The three 'Ps' of interdisciplinary teamwork

Effective interdisciplinary teamwork requires structures that promote collective commitment to quality care. Such interprofessional work encompasses the three 'Ps' of:

- philosophy;
- policy; and
- patient.

    In working with other professionals, nurses must therefore:

- be explicit about their *philosophy* and values;
- participate in *policy* generation that promotes interprofessional cooperation; and
- engage in research and dialogue that places the *patient* at the centre of care delivery.

Nursing values and practices

In playing their part in such interdisciplinary structures, nurses and nurse managers must articulate a coherent philosophy of care. However, nurses have traditionally been reluctant to engage in the more public areas of hospital or healthcare life (West & Scott 2000). Several strategies for making nursing concerns and practices known to other disciplines can be considered. These include:

▶ instituting nursing-led patient rounds;

▶ displaying nursing research in highly visible locations;

▶ implementing multidisciplinary clinical supervision;

▶ arranging shared educational endeavours;

▶ promoting teamwork through social activities, gatherings, and shared tea and meal breaks; and

▶ developing a culture of pride in nursing work.

    Each of these is discussed below.

Instituting nursing-led patient rounds

If carefully planned and conducted by an articulate nurse manager, *nursing-led patient rounds* can showcase nursing skills in the overall context of service delivery. The nurse manager can acknowledge the work of others and, at the same time, demonstrate the specific knowledge and skills of nurses.

Other nurses in attendance can be inspired and learn through the example of a good leader.

Displaying nursing research in highly visible locations

Research papers are of little value to anyone if they remain hidden on shelves. Although nurses frequently present their work to other nurses, they do not often share their work with other disciplines. There are several ways for the nurse manager to bring nursing research to the attention of others. These include:

▶ a short presentation in a tea break, staff meeting, or other forum;
▶ an eye-catching poster that succinctly displays the work and the findings of significance; and
▶ a symposium organised to highlight research that pertains to current clinical issues.

If the last option is adopted, it is advisable for the nurse manager to provide guidance to nurses who lack confidence in presentation skills. If the presentation is of low standard, this reflects poorly on both the nurse and profession.

Strategies for promoting nursing values

Several strategies for making nursing concerns and practices known to other disciplines can be considered. These include:

• instituting nursing-led patient rounds;
• displaying nursing research in highly visible locations;
• implementing multidisciplinary clinical supervision;
• arranging shared educational endeavours;
• promoting teamwork through social activities, gatherings, and shared tea and meal breaks; and
• developing a culture of pride in nursing work.

Each of these is discussed in this section of the chapter.

Implementing multidisciplinary clinical supervision

Multidisciplinary group clinical supervision is a good way to reflect on practice from different perspectives. Examination of clinical scenarios in a multidisciplinary setting enables concerns—both shared concerns and those distinctive to a specific discipline—to be identified and discussed.

In such exercises it is important to be tolerant of the diverse opinions of the various healthcare disciplines. If alternative views of optimal care are to be identified, it is essential that all disciplines recognise their common bond of providing optimal care.

Such multidisciplinary clinical groups require nurse managers to arrange dedicated time and service coverage so that staff members can participate.

Arranging shared educational endeavours

Shared educational forums support collaborative learning and exchange. Many clinical issues that involve all disciplines are of great interest, and examination of these issues creates opportunities for examining shared solutions.

Promoting teamwork

Teamwork is enhanced though social activities, gatherings, and shared meal and tea breaks. Marking milestones and achievements by the whole healthcare team through celebration and the sharing of food and drink helps to build camaraderie and facilitates sharing, mutual respect, and bonding.

Developing a culture of pride in nursing work

Professional 'artistry' and 'craft knowledge' are what all healthcare professionals aspire to achieve (Scholes & Vaughan 2002). Nurses are primarily known for their engagement of patients and families, and their knowledge of those in their care.

'If nurses are confident about nursing work and proud of their professional skills, mutual recognition of good nursing practice is enhanced.'

If nurses are confident about nursing work and nursing management and proud of their professional skills, mutual recognition of good nursing practice is enhanced. Nurses are then more likely to display their own skills, and are more likely to recognise nursing-type skills that are displayed by other healthcare practitioners.

Interdisciplinary teamwork strategies
Patient-centred collaboration

In attempting to diminish interdisciplinary conflict, a sound philosophy for the nurse manager to adopt is a focus on the patient—not on the professions. Because patient advocacy has long been a cornerstone of nursing practice, such a patient-focused perspective in interprofessional collaboration provides excellent opportunities for nurses to lead the way.

It is increasingly accepted throughout the world that the delivery and evaluation of health services should be informed by consumers and carers, and nurses are comfortably placed to help other healthcare professionals to cultivate relationships with consumers. The increasing importance of the consumer perspective is a response to the medical disease approach that was discussed earlier (Stuhlmiller 2003). Consumers, as capable and knowledgeable receivers of care, can challenge professionals who might see themselves as the sole holders of expertise. Working collaboratively, nurses and nurse managers can help to dispel these views. Nurses can highlight core values of nursing practice, such as:

- a focus on consumer strengths and achievements;
- learning about the lived experience of consumers and their families; and
- valuing the healing potential in the relationship between consumers and all care providers.

Nursing research

Nursing research can also be brought to the fore by the nurse manager when working interprofessionally towards increased consumer collaboration. Nursing research has tended to focus on human responses to health problems, with less emphasis on the actual disease process itself. Concern for comfort, care, meaning, and quality of life have taken precedence over other concerns—such as quick fixes through technology. Nursing research is thus well placed to emphasise human connections in health systems that are sometimes accused of lacking a commitment to person-centred care.

Strategies for interdisciplinary teamwork

Strategies for improving interdisciplinary teamwork include the following:
- adopting a philosophy of patient-centred collaboration;
- making use of nursing research;
- implementing consumer surveys and feedback; and
- coordinating assessment;
  Each of these is discussed in this section of the chapter.

Consumer surveys and feedback

Nurse managers can also enhance interprofessional work through consumer surveys or care feedback sheets. These have been shown to be useful in enabling patients to identify what they believe to be the contribution of various disciplines to health care. Such surveys can also provide recognition to disciplines that are otherwise unacknowledged.

Coordinating assessment

The number of discipline-specific health assessments that consumers are required to undergo can be excessive. It is tiresome for patients to be asked the same questions repeatedly. Devising a way to conduct a complete 'interprofessional intake history and assessment' would be welcomed by patients and would enable a more comprehensive and shared view of the person.

Interprofessional care and collaboration would also be improved. With a more complete picture, each team member could become clearer on what he or she is contributing to the overall care plan, and support for the work of others would be facilitated.

Conclusion

Differing models of care can drive the perspectives, concerns, and practices of the various professionals who make up a multidisciplinary health team. Tension and conflict can be created among disciplinary groups if something of central importance to the work of a particular group is threatened or blocked.

An understanding of the different perspectives of various groups can open up new ways of thinking about interprofessional work, and can help to generate respect and support for differing views and practices.

The nurse manager is in an ideal position to facilitate the process of working together as a team.

'The nurse manager is in an ideal position to facilitate the process of working together as a team.'

Chapter 6

Making Meetings Work

Sheila Allen

Introduction

Meetings can be an asset or a liability for a busy nurse manager. These gatherings are critical elements in the management of healthcare facilities. Meetings can be held in various settings and can be formal or informal. However, all meetings must have certain key elements if they are to create value for the organisation by defining issues of importance, resolving problems, and making decisions.

Because the nurse manager can spend a great deal of time in meetings, this chapter contains practical advice about these key elements, and presents vital information on how to achieve desired outcomes in managing meetings. Whether the nurse manager is a participant or a facilitator, knowledge of these key elements will assist in utilising meeting time wisely and in improving the nurse manager's ability to manage his or her role with confidence.

Considerations for meetings

Professional meetings almost always use a variation of 'Robert's Rules of Order' (Constitution Society 2003) as a form of procedural authority. This set of useful guidelines will assist with the governance of any meeting. The underlying principles that guide these rules are (Rogers 1993):

◗ justice and courtesy for all;
◗ consideration of a single item of business at a time;
◗ the right of the minority to be heard;
◗ protection for those absent;
◗ partiality to no single group;
◗ the right of the majority to rule;
◗ stipulations as points of order; and
◗ rules for voting.

'A productive meeting brings together the right people, with the right knowledge, for a defined purpose.'

In healthcare settings, regular meetings of various sorts are often held merely by habit, or to get away from daily work. A *productive* meeting brings together the right people, with the right knowledge, for a defined purpose.

Cost should be a pivotal consideration in the planning of any meeting. Calculating the time expended by participants—including planning, preparation of meeting materials, and travel—should be an important factor in determining whether a meeting is needed. To improve the likelihood of success, the purpose of the meeting and how long it should last should be defined, and the attendance of relevant people should be facilitated (Hindle 1998). It should always be remembered that if an issue or problem can be solved or resolved without a meeting, there is no need for that meeting.

The purpose of a meeting might be to deal with information, to resolve an issue or problem, to make decisions, or to encourage ideas in a brainstorming session. Once the need for the meeting has been established, preparation is pivotal to the success of the meeting. Time spent in planning for a meeting is rarely wasted.

Planning elements

The purpose of a meeting will determine the urgency of that meeting. Some of the factors to be considered are:

◗ How many people should attend, and who should they be?
◗ Where, and at what time, should the meeting be held?
◗ Will audiovisual equipment be needed?

‣ Will catering be necessary?
‣ How many breaks will be needed?
‣ What kind of seating will be needed?
‣ What are the desired outcomes?

Once the objectives are defined, it is easier to develop an agenda. The nurse manager might start with an item that will unify the group (Nichols 1998). When planning a meeting, the following points should be considered:

‣ schedule important topics (those that will be most critical to the achievement of expected objectives) towards the beginning of the meeting;
‣ separate the difficult topics;
‣ evaluate realistically the number of topics that can be covered in the established time for the meeting;
‣ state (in the agenda) the date, time, place, and purpose of the meeting, the items for discussion, and the time allocated for discussion of each item;
‣ remember that participants usually do not mind finishing a meeting early, but meetings that run over the expected time frustrate many people;
‣ circulate the draft agenda to the invited participants and request their input;
‣ incorporate any suggestions of those attending into another draft of the agenda and recirculate the final draft;
‣ ensure that all materials required for effective discussion are distributed before the meeting, so that participants have time to prepare for knowledge-based discussion and decision-making; and
‣ ensure that participants are aware that they are expected to review the material and to notify the chair if they are unable to attend.

The agenda is a list of the issues to be discussed and debated. It is therefore a 'blueprint' of the meeting, and should be as short and simple as possible. Figure 6.1 (page 62) is an example of an agenda.

One tool that the chair can employ to expedite business is a general *consent vote* or *consent agenda*. A consent vote can include a number of related items (such as committee reports). This approach should never be employed if the issue is serious or controversial (Denholm 1998). The chair must first ascertain that the matter is acceptable to all. The chair should ask for any objection, and then state the business on which the consent vote will be taken. If any participant objects, each item must be considered separately. If there is no objection, the motion can be considered and the vote taken.

Executive Committee Meeting

23 June, 9.30 am

Texas Room, Random Hotel
1. 9:30   Call to order; establish quorum
2. 9:35   Minutes
3. 9:40   Financial
4. 9:50   Reports from committees
5. 10:10   Correspondence
6. 10:15   Break
7. 10:25   Unfinished business
             (i) Review Correct Site Policy
             (ii) Regulatory requirement review (history and physicals
             on chart)
8. 10:45   Other business
9. 10:55   Review meeting
             Prepare next meeting assignments
10. 11:00   Adjournment

Figure 6.1 Sample agenda
Author's creation

Keeping order

As outlined above, most meetings utilise some form of accepted procedural protocol, such as 'Robert's Rules of Order' (Constitution Society 2003). The use of such an authority can significantly shorten the length of the meeting, increase productivity, and reduce friction among participants. If the nurse manager is not familiar with such procedures, a library or the Internet can be consulted for guidance (Constitution Society 2003). Such procedural protocols can be adapted to fit the needs of any meeting and any organisation. They are flexible, provide democracy and equity, protect the rights of all participants, and provide for a fair hearing for all. Participants 'have their say' by presenting, debating, and voting on motions. Most importantly, the procedure provides a means of maintaining courtesy at all times.

> 'Protocols are flexible, provide democracy and equity, protect the rights of all, and provide for a fair hearing.'

To facilitate business and accomplish agreed outcomes participants must:
▶ be recognised by the chair before speaking;
▶ present motions that are in order;

▶ speak clearly and concisely; and
▶ obey rules of debate and discussion.

In addition, procedural rules for the meeting should be established and distributed to participants before the meeting. Some examples of such procedural rules are:

▶ set the time for beginning and adjournment;
▶ establish discussion times for each agenda item;
▶ require all remarks to be made through the chair (to discourage private conversations);
▶ alternate between speakers who are 'for' and 'against' a motion;
▶ set the length of time someone may speak;
▶ limit the number of times a person may speak before all have spoken; and
▶ state the number of times a person may speak on any one issue.

When rules are established and communicated before the meeting, the chair can avoid the pitfalls associated with domineering behaviour, and can ensure that respectful dialogue enhances the proceedings.

Getting things done

Behaviour of participants

To facilitate business and accomplish agreed outcomes participants must:
• be recognised by the chair before speaking;
• present motions that are in order;
• speak clearly and concisely; and
• obey rules of debate and discussion.

Procedural rules

Procedural rules should:
• set the time for beginning and adjournment;
• establish discussion times for each agenda item;
• require all remarks to be made through the chair (to discourage private conversations);
• alternate between speakers who are 'for' and 'against' a motion;
• set the length of time someone may speak;
• limit the number of times a person may speak before all have spoken; and
• state the number of times a person may speak on any one issue.

Attention should also be paid to the terms of reference for a meeting—that is, a description of why the meeting is being held. For example, a committee might meet on a regular basis to debate issues affecting the nursing staff of the

LIVERPOOL JOHN MOORES UNIVERSITY
LEARNING & INFORMATION SERVICES

surgical suite and to offer suggestions for their management. Another committee might be called to discuss the high level of absenteeism and casual sickness in a particular nursing team. Establishing the clear terms of reference for a meeting ensures that the purpose of the meeting is clearly defined.

Effective environment

Ideally, the nurse manager has some control of the location and seating arrangements for the meeting. To facilitate a successful meeting, some general rules for seating are (Hindle 1998):

▶ participants should not be seated in direct sunlight;
▶ participants should be seated at least an arm's length apart;
▶ participants should be able to see and be seen; and
▶ chairs that are too comfortable should be avoided.

The seating arrangement might vary in accordance with cultural differences, confronting opinions, tactical strategies, or the need to create an atmosphere for open discussion. In some cultures, factors such as age, station, and position might require that the seating arrangements reflect the appropriate hierarchy for the occasion. If there are negotiations or opposing views, participants can be seated around a rectangular table with participants who hold opposing views facing each other. However, it is not always appropriate that all people with the same view sit on either side; alternating seating can provide a more neutral forum. For free and open discussion, a round table provides a more equitable seating arrangement.

All participants should listen respectfully to others, be aware of negative body language, avoid irrelevant debate, and present ideas clearly, succinctly, and positively.

Chairing and facilitating a meeting

The chair or facilitator fulfils the important role of ensuring that the meeting runs smoothly, that the proceedings are directed, and that desired objectives are met. Because this person has usually done all the planning, created the agenda, arranged for the necessary equipment and catering, and invited the participants, he or she is the person most familiar with the objectives. Before the meeting, the chair should study the agenda, plan the order, and become familiar with the participants.

Responsibility for the progression and good order of the meeting lies with the chair. The chair should:

- start and end on time;
- ensure that documentation of the meeting is completed;
- synthesise and summarise points clearly and succinctly;
- be flexible in dealing with the different styles of participants;
- be open and receptive, and encourage participation by all;
- ensure that all sides of issues are explored in a respectful manner;
- block any negative tactics used by participants;
- ensure that voting is properly handled; and
- cast the determining vote when necessary.

It is the responsibility of the chair to pace the meeting so that it remains on track and on time. However, the chair should refrain from stating his or her opinion because these remarks can unduly influence participants or prevent participants from expressing their views. If the pace is lagging, the chair might consider skipping non-essential parts of the agenda. He or she needs to obtain the agreement of all before taking this course of action. By keeping to the agenda and strictly maintaining time limits, the chair can ensure that time is efficiently managed.

An appropriate duration of time before a scheduled break is 90 minutes (Hindle 1998). If the meeting is scheduled to run for two hours, a break can be offered or planned after one hour. A break can also be utilised to deal directly with behaviour that is disruptive. A word of caution spoken privately to the participant concerned can help to alleviate the problem.

Although the chair's task is to keep the group focused, he or she should avoid talking too much. To ensure that all participants have an opportunity to make their points, the chair should develop some method of monitoring speakers.

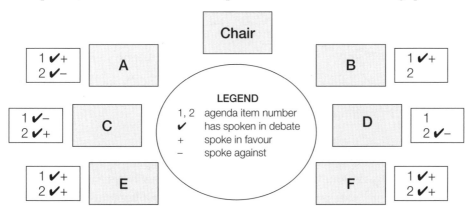

Figure 6.2 Monitoring by doodles
Author's creation

Because participants might raise their hands to be recognised by the chair, a list of names in order of recognition can provide a helpful means of keeping order. By a method of doodling (see Figure 6.2, page 65), the chair can keep track of who has spoken, the number of times that person has spoken, and his or her position on an issue. Numbered agenda items can be helpful in modifying the method to enable the chair to monitor many phases of discussion. Use of any method takes practice, so each chairperson must find the method that works best for him or her.

To facilitate the meeting, the chair should periodically restate the issue under discussion, and summarise discussion. The objective is to seek consensus, but not necessarily to have everyone agree. In seeking consensus, the group searches for a solution that all participants can support, even if individual members do not agree with every facet of the proposal.

Handling difficult participants

If there is a disruption during the meeting, the chair must deal with the problem swiftly and efficiently. The rules for the meeting that are circulated before the meeting provide a basis for all actions by the chair.

Certain behaviours by participants can escalate or become slanderous. The most efficient ways to defuse disruptive behaviours are to guide the participants back to the discussion at hand, to call for a vote, or to call for a break.

Most people who participate in a meeting are interested in a positive outcome and achieving the goals of the meeting. Meetings proceed efficiently when all are prepared to participate in such a positive manner. Sometimes the easiest way to change the atmosphere of a meeting is to change the subject. Whatever method is utilised, the chair must take control of the situation and then move on in a positive fashion.

'Sometimes the easiest way to change the atmosphere of a meeting is to change the subject.'

Closing the meeting

Once the business is completed, the chair brings the meeting to a close. This is the time, while all participants are available for consultation, to summarise discussion, recap decisions, organise assignments (if needed), and arrange for the next meeting. When the chair summarises the meeting, any issues that require additional discussion should be highlighted.

Meetings should always end on a positive note, with all participants being thanked for their contributions to the discussion. All opinions enrich the dialogue. If participants know that their time is appreciated, they are more likely to continue to be actively involved in continuing dialogue and resolving issues that arise in the future.

An evaluation tool can be distributed to participants with a request that they fill them out before departing.

Follow-up action between meetings

The responsibilities of the chair or facilitator do not end when the meeting is adjourned. Minutes or notes from the meeting should be reviewed and sent to all participants in a timely manner (Nichols 1998). Distribution can usually be accomplished within a week's time. Participants should be notified when they can expect a report of the meeting. Decisions that require action should be clearly defined in the notes or in a separate report so that there is no confusion regarding assignments. Between meetings, the chair might ask participants to send progress reports that can be shared with the group to keep everyone on task and informed.

An assessment or evaluation is just as important to the success of the meeting as it is to patient care. A tool that asks pertinent questions of participants and provides rating options is a simple way of finding out how the participants perceived the meeting. Questions that might be effective are:

▶ Were the agenda items pertinent?
▶ Was the overall meeting effective?
▶ Was appropriate time spent on agenda items?
▶ What would you change about the meeting?

With a few questions, and space for comments, positive results can be achieved. There are resources for assessment tools to benchmark performance and access information (Partridge 2000). A review of the evaluation tool can yield information that can be utilised to identify points that might improve future meetings.

Conference call meeting

As meetings and facilities become more sophisticated, business might be conducted by conference call. There might be a need to address an issue between the regularly scheduled meetings, and a conference call is often a more efficient way to conduct such interim business. Because conference calls do not involve eye contact, the individual environments of participants can distract them more easily, and attention spans are therefore not as long. The chair of a conference-call meeting must be skilled at steering discussions to keep participants focused on the subject at hand. This type of meeting requires a greater degree of preparation.

As with other meetings, the chair must schedule the time and date for the call and must coordinate all participants. Because the call should be no more than one hour (Schlegel 2000), a brief agenda is vital to the success of the meeting. The resource materials and agenda should be sent to participants 48–72 hours before the call (Chang 1992). Like other meetings, the call should start and end on time. Participants should be welcomed and asked to state their names each time they speak. If remarks are unclear, the chair can assist participants with questions or comments—such as: 'Could you give an example, please?'. Shorter comments usually keep attention focused and the energy of the participants heightened. Frequent summary and efficient follow-up are just as important for a conference call as they are for ordinary meetings. As the time draws to a close, the chair should review accomplishments, thank participants, and plan for the next meeting.

Conclusion

Nurse managers are busy, efficient people who know how to guide, stimulate, probe, and mediate; they do it every day. These skills can facilitate meetings and contribute to their success. By the application of some basic principles, nurse managers can add real value to meetings.

'Planning is the key to the success of any meeting.'

Planning is the key to the success of any meeting. Apart from preparation and practice, the following principles apply to presiding over a meeting (Schlegel 1994):

- ▶ start on time;
- ▶ announce the purpose and goals of the meeting and how the agenda items relate;
- ▶ restate a motion before calling for a vote;
- ▶ ensure that all issues come to a fair vote;
- ▶ validate the vote;
- ▶ organise assignments based on required action;
- ▶ keep to the agenda and encourage participation by all; and
- ▶ end the meeting on time.

An important element is to appreciate participation, given the busy schedule of many people. For the nurse manager, practice will provide the confidence needed to participate in and conduct meetings that accomplish goals, provide solutions, and encourage participation.

Chapter 7

Counselling Your Staff

Andrew Crowther

Introduction

When a staff member comes to a nurse manager for counselling, that staff member expects to take part in a confidential, skilled interview through which he or she hopes to feel better and receive help in solving problems (Geldard & Geldard 2001). Counselling staff involves skilled intervention, confidentiality, and, most importantly, the ability to help staff members find a solution to their problems. Counselling is not a pleasant chat between friends; rather, it is a structured attempt to provide help in a problem situation.

Counselling, if undertaken properly, is never neutral. When a nurse manager spends time in a counselling relationship with a staff member, something in the life of that staff member will change; that person's ability to explore, cope, and solve problems will be enhanced or diminished (Egan 1998).

> 'Counselling staff involves skilled intervention, confidentiality, and the ability to help staff members find a solution to their problems.'

The complexity of staff counselling

Because the employer–employee relationship is based on authority, seniority, and power imbalance, counselling staff is more complex than many other counselling relationships. The nurse–client relationship crosses fewer hierarchical boundaries, and it is easier to keep within accepted norms for those roles. Counselling staff, especially if the staff member works in the nurse manager's immediate team, is more limited in terms of the depth of self revealed by both manager and employee, and in the range of outcomes that might result from the counselling session.

Staff counselling should not be disciplinary in nature. Taking action against an employee for some incorrect practice falls outside the remit of the counsellor's role. A nurse manager might, of course, be otherwise involved in disciplining a staff member—together with professional organisations and human resources personnel. However, such a disciplinary role is *not* counselling. Misunderstanding this basic distinction has given rise to the misplaced assertion: 'Oh yes, I severely counselled her about that'.

Similarly, counselling is not the same thing as performance appraisal or individual performance review. Those important interventions with staff, which are discussed in Chapter 12 of this book, are also separate from the counselling relationship. However, nurse managers might well be involved in counselling a staff member who has performed poorly during an appraisal. It is important in such circumstances that the manager finds reasons for staff members functioning at less than their ideal level, but this involves an interview (or a series of interviews) that are quite separate from the appraisal.

'Counselling is not the same thing as performance appraisal or individual performance review.'

Possible conflicts

Nurse managers who are attempting to counsel their staff will encounter areas of potential conflict. Many nurses perceive counselling as something that falls outside the role of the nurse and of the nurse manager. Counselling seems to have become 'owned' by other disciplines. However, counselling is actually a key component of nursing management and an important aspect of interacting with colleagues and patients alike.

Apart from this perception that counselling is 'not done' by nurses, nurse managers can also face problems if organisational goals and culture are defined *for* the nurse manager. Beliefs and actions, at least in public, are often prescribed for the nurse manager by his or her superiors. This can cause problems. A nurse manager who wants to work with his or her staff as people, and not as disposable resources, will not find life easy within an organisation that values only the meeting of budget deadlines. However, it is self-evident that a competent nurse

'Counselling is a key component of nursing management and an important aspect of interacting with colleagues and patients alike.'

manager must be able to work with people as the single most important component of the health-care delivery system. Counselling staff is central to any understanding of working effectively with people.

The nature of the counselling relationship

When counselling staff, the nurse manager will be dealing with work-related problems that affect the employee. These are likely to involve:

▶ family;
▶ rostering and shift problems;
▶ colleagues;
▶ job stress (especially post-trauma);
▶ various other work-related issues (such as examinations, visas, work permits, and registration issues); and
▶ issues external to work (such as illness).

Whatever the issue confronting the employee, the nurse manager has to adopt the appropriate role of a counsellor. This involves being:

▶ courteous;
▶ non-threatening;
▶ non-authoritarian; and
▶ safe.

It is not easy to adopt such a role. Nursing tends to be hierarchical and authoritarian, with carefully delineated lines of accountability and reporting. Indeed, many nurses stay in the profession because they gain comfort from the psychological safety of such relationships, and it can be difficult for the nurse manager to step outside these hierarchical stereotypes in which the person being counselled is perceived as a junior who must respect the position and wisdom of the nurse manager.

The term 'safe' in the list above refers to the crafting of a relationship in which the person being counselled feels able to share his or her concerns—

without fear of being ridiculed, belittled, or denied any prospects of promotion. If staff members fear disciplinary action or punishment, they will not come to the nurse manager in the first instance.

The complexity of employer–employee counselling is increased when the circumstances of the initial request for a counselling interview are considered. Did the nurse manager ask the nurse to come? Did the nurse come of his or her own volition? Did another nurse think that there might be something to be gained if the employee came to see the nurse manager?

'Coming to see a nurse manager at all can involve high personal cost for the employee.'

It must be remembered that coming to see a nurse manager at all can involve high personal cost for the employee. When word gets out that a junior nurse has been to the manager, this can have a negative effect on:

- the opinions of the junior nurse's peers and colleagues (especially because nurses like to see themselves as 'coping', no matter what happens);
- the nurse manager's opinion of the junior nurse (if only in the perception of the employee);
- the cohesion and effectiveness of the nursing team;
- the stress level experienced by the junior nurse (who might have a self-perception of having failed because he or she needed to come to the nurse manager in the first instance); and
- the nurse manager's relationship with the staff member (in view of the power imbalance between the respective positions).

All of these elements can increase stress for the employee, and it is therefore important to praise him or her for being there, and for having the courage to come and see the nurse manager.

Apart from generating problems for the person being counselled, there can also be problems for the nurse manager. These might relate to the nurse manager:

- not seeing counselling as a legitimate part of the nurse-management role;
- feeling underprepared and unskilled;
- not really wanting to get involved; or
- having no real interest in the well-being of staff.

Methods of counselling

There are many models of counselling that can be used. Most adhere to a basic humanistic approach, and most cover much the same ground. The following is a model that the present author has evolved over a period of time and which has proven to be useful in various counselling settings. The model takes account of the important parameters of environment, self, time, and outcomes (ESTO). Each of these elements is discussed below.

Environment

The environment in which the nurse manager decides to counsel is of central importance to the success of the interview. Although it is difficult to find quiet areas in many hospitals or health-care facilities, a meaningful interview cannot take place if there is undue extraneous noise. The nurse manager should choose an area in which the interview will not be interrupted by telephones, pagers, or knocks at the door. A 'neutral' venue should be chosen. The nurse manager might be comfortable in his or her own office—with its familiar props, piles of important-looking folders, and packed bookcases—but the employee is unlikely to be comfortable in such a setting.

> 'The environment in which the nurse manager decides to counsel is of central importance to the success of the interview.'

Seating is also important. The participants should be seated at the same level—preferably in low chairs placed a metre or so apart, and turned towards each other at an angle of about 45 degrees. The employee should be offered the choice of chairs, and care should be taken to allow him or her to sit between the nurse manager and the door. This minimises the possibility of the employee feeling trapped or constrained. Indeed, some nurse managers will not counsel with the door closed. Although this does present problems with confidentiality, this approach helps to ensure a greater measure of psychological freedom for the person being counselled.

There should not be a clock in view. It is likely that the counsellor's eyes will be irresistibly drawn to it, and this can indicate to the employee that the nurse manager is bored and wants to finish the session.

Any table should be low so that it does not form a physical barrier between the participants. An 'engaged' sign should be placed outside the door, and instructions should be given that the conversation is not to be disturbed.

Self

The nurse manager should be aware of how he or she is presenting to the employee. The manager should be relaxed, with his or her body angled towards the employee in an 'open posture'. There should be no folding of arms, hugging of files or clipboards to the chest, or any other body language that might signal 'closed'. The nurse manager should avoid turning away from the conversation at any time, because this might be interpreted as indicating a lack of interest. Similarly, putting up the feet, or eating lunch, can indicate a lack of involvement.

The manager should try to maintain eye contact with the staff member. It is important not to stare, challenge, or show disgust or incredulity. It is also important to be aware that different cultures attach various social meanings to eye contact (Egan 1988).

It is helpful to attempt to validate what the employee is saying by using non-verbal and para-verbal communication. The giving of an affirmative nod or an occasional murmur of 'Uh-huh' might seem to be simplistic, but both are very effective in communicating positive reinforcement.

The interview should begin with the nurse manager focusing on the person, and not the facts of the matter. Before focusing on the specific issue at hand, it is important to spend some time 'being with' the person, thanking him or her for coming, and finding out how this person is feeling and what is happening to him or her at this time.

The aim is to achieve what Geldard and Geldard (2001) have termed a 'two person just society'—a meeting of two people that is not tainted by the sort of power imbalance in which one person is exposed, unwillingly, to personal self-examination by the other. As far as possible, the aim is equality in the counselling relationship.

If difficulties are experienced in getting the session moving, it can be useful to repeat part of any statement that the employee might have used to start the conversation. For example, the employee might have been prepared to venture: 'I'm not coping on the ward at the moment'. The nurse manager can reply: 'Not coping . . .?'. This might seem crass and simplistic, but it is very effective in encouraging a person to open up and begin to share problems.

The ESTO model of staff counselling

The ESTO model discussed in this chapter takes account of the important parameters of: (i) environment; (ii) self; (iii) time; and (iv) outcomes. The important elements of the model can be summarised as follows.

Environment
- quiet areas and no undue extraneous noise
- an area in which the interview will not be interrupted
- a 'neutral' venue

(continued)

(Continued)
- attention to seating, doors, tables, clocks, and so on
- an 'engaged' sign placed outside the door, and instructions given that the conversation is not to be disturbed

Self
- awareness of how the nurse manager is presenting to the employee
- relaxed, 'open' posture; no body language that might signal 'closed'
- avoid turning away from the conversation at any time; avoid any suggestion of lack of interest
- maintain eye contact, but be aware that different cultures attach various social meaning to eye contact
- validate by using non-verbal and para-verbal communication
- begin by focusing on the person, and not the facts of the matter
- aim for a 'two person just society', with equality in the counselling relationship
- validate comments by repetition of part of what has been said

Time
- decide how much time can be devoted to the counselling session
- time must be uninterrupted
- share time constraints quite openly
- impart a sense of getting down to business and not just chatting in a pleasant, aimless way
- if subsequent appointment is made, adhere to time, day, and place agreed

Outcomes
- work together towards outcomes that are realistic and achievable
- shared strategies (not merely a suggestion of the nurse manager which the employee feels pressured into adopting)
- all possible ways forward considered
- strategy written down succinctly
- seek outside assistance if required
- definite timeframe for achievable outcomes incorporated into joint discussions and planning
- focus initially on short-term achievable goals
- employee record of what has been achieved

Time

Before beginning, the nurse manager must decide how much time can be devoted to the counselling session. As noted above, this must be *uninterrupted* time.

At the beginning of the interview, it is wise to share the time constraints quite openly: 'OK, I have about forty minutes to share with you; then I really have to be at another meeting. Until then, my time's all yours.' This approach demonstrates that the nurse manager values the person, and has made time for him or her alone. It also puts a reasonable timeframe around the session and imparts a sense of getting down to business—not just chatting in a pleasant, aimless way. Once the time has been set, it is important that the timeframe be observed by both parties.

Similarly, if it is decided that another meeting is needed with this person, and if a subsequent appointment is made, it is important that the nurse manager adheres to the time, day, and place agreed.

Outcomes

There is little point in spending time together in an interview if there is no outcome other than a pleasant chat. If a plan to move things forward is not crafted together, both the nurse manager and the employee are wasting their time. There is a need to work together towards outcomes. These outcomes should be realistic and achievable. To ensure this, possible strategies should be explored with the employee. Such strategies should not merely be a suggestion of the nurse manager which the employee feels pressured into adopting.

Working with the employee, all possible ways forward should be considered—however outrageous or far-fetched each idea might seem at first. Each idea should then be worked through, with the strengths and weaknesses of each one being considered. When there is mutual agreement on which outcome is the best to follow, and when the nurse manager is sure that this is the *employee's* own choice (and not the one that he or she feels that the *nurse manager* wants to follow), the strategy should be written down succinctly.

'All possible ways forward should be considered—however outrageous or far-fetched each idea might seem at first.'

The strategies that the staff member is going to utilise as he or she works towards the chosen outcome should then be summarised. Of these outcomes, some will be achievable before the next meeting (for example, making an appointment to see a colleague to discuss an area of personal conflict, or enquiring about a move to a community-based team), whereas others will take longer (for example, applying for a place on a master's degree course). In some cases it might be mutually agreed that there is a need to seek outside assistance, perhaps in the form of a referral to another health professional.

The timeframe to be applied to these achievable outcomes must also be incorporated into the joint discussions and planning.

It is best to focus initially on short-term achievable goals. Attaining these will afford a sense of progress for the employee, and will allow him or her to feel that something is being achieved in regaining control over his or her own affairs. Assessment of the level of such success then becomes the starting-point for the next interview. If there is a range of different strategies to be followed before the next interview, it is useful if the employee keeps a record of what he or she has achieved. This is best done in the form of a diary—perusal of which can be the first phase of the next session.

Issues to be considered

Beware of filters

When counselling, the nurse manager should be on the look out for 'filters'. Just as a filter on a camera lens affects what is seen, a nurse manager is sometimes unable to see and hear a staff member without the manager's preconceptions and value judgments colouring or 'filtering' impressions. These filters might be preconceptions regarding culture, professional standing, expertise, gender, universities, specialities, and so on.

Filters might also be based on the nurse manager's previous experience of a particular staff member or that person's place of work. The manager might feel:

▶ 'She always copes, this must be somebody else's fault.'
▶ 'Here we are again, another problem from the night shift on the surgical ward.'
▶ 'Mental health nurses should be able to cope with these things themselves.'

Each of these sorts of preconceptions will prevent the nurse manager objectively assessing the person and the situation, and the counselling session will thus be rendered less effective. The nurse manager must consciously put aside his or her pre-conceptions. These preconceptions must, in effect, be placed 'in brack-ets' so that they do not cause bias in making a proper assessment of the situation.

> 'The nurse manager must consciously put aside preconceptions.'

Importance of first interview

A nurse manager might find that a staff member undertakes the first interview merely to establish the nurse manager's credentials as a counsellor and to see if confidentiality is maintained. In these circumstances, the staff member might share only a small part of the problem, no matter how skilled the nurse manager is in getting people to open up and share. There will then be a pause before the employee comes back again—while he or she waits to see if confidential information comes back by gossip from other members of staff. If this should happen, the nurse manager will lose all credibility as a counsellor with that employee. Moreover, it is likely that other employees will also lose confidence and the nurse manager will find a significant decrease in the number of people coming for counselling.

Apart from the question of confidentiality, the first interview might also be used by an employee to see how good the nurse manager is at counselling, and whether he or she actually does what is promised. A problem often encountered by nurses who make an appointment to see their manager is that they do not encounter the sensitive counsellor they expected. Rather, they find themselves confronted by a senior staff member who wants to shut them up and get them back to work as quickly as possible. Managers who see their employees as resources to be exploited, rather than as human beings to be nurtured and valued, are unlikely to make competent counsellors.

'Managers who see their employees as resources to be exploited, rather than as human beings to be nurtured and valued, are unlikely to make competent counsellors.'

Using other counsellors

Some organisations employ their own 'staff counsellor'. Employees are referred to this person, or ask to be referred to this person. This can be an effective arrangement, but it can be fraught with problems—the most common of which is the issue of confidentiality. The nurse manager is then dependent on being informed of the outcome of an interview between the nurse manager's staff member and the designated counsellor. This can lead to a breakdown of trust and a decrease in utilisation of the counselling service.

Another option is for the employing authority to contract an outside counsellor to provide a counselling service to staff. A staff member might be referred to that counsellor for a series of confidential counselling sessions. In this scenario, the staff member uses his or her manager as an access point for counselling, rather than for the counselling itself. This arrangement has budgetary implications because, when the series of counselling sessions is finished, the account is often sent to the manager for re-imbursement.

Confidentiality can also be an issue in this arrangement. Because the nurse manager pays for the service, he or she might presume, incorrectly, to have a right to know what the employee has been discussing in confidential counselling with an external counsellor.

Supervision

Every nurse manager who undertakes counselling should consider the issue of counselling supervision. The problems and concerns that staff members share with their manager can accumulate, and these can impact on the nurse manager as well as on staff members involved. As a nurse manager gains credibility as a counsellor, and as more people attend, this accumulation of problems can become increasingly burdensome. A nurse manager who undertakes counselling should therefore carefully select someone to act as the manager's supervisor.

Because of the power imbalances that are inherent in hospitals and health professions, it is not a good idea to have the manager's professional senior as a counselling supervisor. Ideally, the counselling supervisor should be of the same grade as the counsellor—perhaps with a little more experience in counselling. The supervisor might be employed by another hospital or health service. This ensures that there is some emotional and professional detachment from the issues at hand.

'Ideally, the counselling supervisor should be of the same grade as the counsellor—perhaps with a little more experience in counselling.'

In working with a counselling supervisor, the nurse manager should:

- set up frequent meetings (at least once per month);
- describe the range of people being seen, but always maintain anonymity;
- explore the strategies being used;
- discuss any problems being experienced with specific approaches;
- allow the supervisor to comment on how he or she perceives the nurse manager's counselling performance;
- allow the supervisor to suggest other strategies that might be employed to make the counselling even more effective; and
- take time outside supervision sessions to reflect on what has been shared, with a view to modifying the counselling approach.

The nurse manager should bear in mind that the relationship with the counselling supervisor is a supportive exercise. This is not the place for a stout defence of what has been done. Rather, this is a constructive exploration in which the goal is the well-being and effectiveness of the nurse manager as counsellor.

The relationship with the counselling supervisor enables the nurse manager to validate his or her skills and effectiveness as a counsellor. In addition, sharing some of the counselling experiences lifts a little of the burden of being a counsellor.

Conclusion

The strategies and hints contained in this chapter will help to ensure that nurse managers who undertake counselling of their staff are effective and ethical in the role.

An ongoing relationship with a counselling supervisor will ensure that the nurse manager maintains high standards and shares some of the burden.

'Nurse managers are being granted an important privilege by those who confidently share their problems with them.'

Finally, nurse managers should always be aware that they are being granted an important privilege by those who confidently share their problems with them.

Chapter 8

Dealing with Unhelpful Nurses

Michael Cully

Introduction

It has never been an easy task to manage workers in healthcare settings. High levels of stress caused by unsociable working hours, together with the emotionally, physically, and intellectually draining nature of clinical-care delivery, have contributed to 'unhelpful' behaviours by nurses.

Recent changes in working conditions have compounded the manager's problems with unhelpful behaviours. For example, the 'mania' for downsizing has increased uncertainty about employment, and the increased use of contract/casual staff and the reduction in permanent/core staff has weakened the organisational culture. Whereas, in the past, there has been a reasonable expectation that employees would understand the organisation's philosophy, policies, and procedures with respect to care delivery, the situation is now less clear. Moreover, the

> 'Recent changes in working conditions have compounded the manager's problems with unhelpful behaviours.'

creation of work teams that have both permanent staff and contract/casual staff has given rise to a number of problem behaviours. These include distrust and stereotyping (Clarke 2003).

Although this chapter deals with specific instances of unhelpful behaviour, the nurse manager should keep the bigger picture in mind. Workloads have increased dramatically, and this has led to heightened stress and greater anger in the workforce (Johnson & Indvik 2001). In addition, the impact of information technologies is being felt in increasing fragmentation of the work group into smaller, semi-autonomous teams. This latter trend has a negative impact upon the development of organisational 'citizenship'—in that workers have fewer opportunities to see themselves as part of a larger organisation. This is amplified when the teams are engaged in short-term projects, and members therefore do not have time to bond as a work group.

Describing unhelpfulness

Nurses can exhibit unhelpful behaviours as *clinicians*, *collaborators*, and *managers*. Each of these is discussed below.

Unhelpful clinical behaviours

Unhelpful clinical behaviours include:
- failure to manage resources and people effectively;
- failure to provide emotional support;
- failure to provide comfort (including adequate analgesia);
- failure to provide correct or adequate information and advice;
- failure to perform technical duties; and
- breaching confidentiality.

Nurses exhibiting unhelpfulness

Nurses can exhibit unhelpful behaviours as:
- clinicians;
- collaborators; and
- managers.

Each of these categories is explored in greater detail in the text of this chapter.

Unhelpful behaviours towards colleagues

Unhelpful behaviours towards colleagues can be 'lumped together' as, simply, 'bullying'. Bullying seems to thrive in an organisational atmosphere of uncertainty in which there is a lack of clear role definition (Archer 1999). Such bullying can be quite open, or it can be remarkably subtle. If overt bullying behaviour attracts

'Bullying can be quite open, or it can be remarkably subtle.'

unfavourable responses from management, it can often reappear in less visible ways (Crawford 1999).

Some of the more obvious forms of bullying include:
▶ physical and verbal assaults;
▶ overt sexual harassment; and
▶ ridiculing others in public.

Some of the less overt forms of bullying include (Hannabuss 1998):
▶ rumour-mongering and gossiping;
▶ isolating the person in the workforce; and
▶ some forms of manipulation.

Unhelpful behaviours as a manager

An unhelpful manager can display the following behaviours (Elangovan 2002):
▶ inappropriate delegation;
▶ setting impossible dates for completion of work;
▶ avoiding taking corrective actions with respect to unhelpful staff behaviours; and
▶ inappropriate interventions with regard to staff behaviours.

Dealing with unhelpful behaviours
Dealing with the unhelpful clinician

If a clinician is displaying unhelpful behaviours, the manager should not put off dealing with the issue—such as waiting until an annual performance review falls due. Problems of unhelpful behaviour will not go away; indeed they might become entrenched (Christie & Kleiner 2000).

If the problems are motivational or relate to people not meeting work standards, it is probably better, in the first instance, to take a personal counselling approach—rather than contemplating disciplinary action. If the behaviours are not major breaches of organisational policy or examples of insubordination, the following approaches can be taken by the manager (Rees 1997).
▶ Set standards that are unambiguous and expressed in behavioural terms.
▶ Allow the employee to state his or her case without interruption in a safe environment.

▶ Suspend judgment until all relevant evidence is available.
▶ Set in train corrective actions (which will usually involve in-house training).
▶ Keep accurate records.

Most of these steps are self-evident. However, the issues surrounding the tendency of some managers to take a *judgmental attitude* are worthy of further exploration.

In assessing judgmental behaviour by managers, it must be recognised that a manager's choice of interventions is influenced by (Elangoven 2002):

▶ the characteristics of the problem behaviour;
▶ the characteristics of people exhibiting or reporting the problem behaviour; and
▶ the characteristics of the manager.

Decisions are influenced by biases and mental shortcuts called 'heuristics'.

Biases can include giving more weight to reports from certain people. For example, a manager might give more credence to reports from core staff than those from casual staff; or the manager might place more value on a report from personal friends and professional colleagues, rather than those of clients or visitors.

Commonly used *heuristics* include 'availability' and 'representativeness'. The *availability* heuristic relies upon the ease with which an instance of an event can be brought to mind. If the manager can easily bring to mind an instance in which the reported behaviour has occurred, it is more likely that the manager will believe that the behaviour is common and might have occurred again in this instance. Consider the example of a clinician being accused of handling a client roughly. If the clinician's manager can readily recollect instances of rough treatment by this person in the past, the manager is more likely to believe that the clinician is guilty (Tversky & Kahneman 1982). The *representativeness* heuristic is used to help solve classification problems—but does so through a form of stereotyping. The manager using this heuristic might be confronted with a report that a mental-health nurse has handled a client roughly. If the manager believes that the potential to be rough is a common characteristic among mental-health nurses, this particular nurse is likely to be considered guilty before the nurse has even presented his or her case.

Managers should not be swayed by bias or rely on heuristic devices to create a false air of certainty about the staff behavioural problems with which they deal.

Judgmental behaviour

Managers can exhibit judgmental behaviour if decisions are influenced by:
- biases; or
- heuristics

Biases include giving more weight to reports from certain people:
- core staff rather than casual staff;
- personal friends and professional colleagues rather than clients or visitors.

Heuristics include:
- availability (easily recalling similar past events); and
- representativeness (stereotyping).

All of these features of judgmental behaviour by managers are explored in greater detail in this section of the text.

Dealing with a major issue

Most infractions of practice or discipline are minor, and these can be dealt with through counselling or mentoring. There is usually no need for a formal process to be implemented. Formal disciplinary processes are time-consuming and often unsettling for workers who are not immediate parties to the situation. It can be

> 'It can be more productive to use the 'velvet glove' rather than the 'mailed fist'.

more productive to use the 'velvet glove' rather than the 'mailed fist'!

However, serious breaches of practice or discipline must be dealt with through formal means. Every healthcare facility or service should have a formal procedure, and managers should adhere to this.

The manager should arrange to meet with the worker whose performance is problematic. The meeting must be private and conducted with an assurance of confidentiality—which means that only those people in the organisation with a legitimate reason will be informed of what is said at the meeting. It is quite common for the person who is the subject of a complaint to be accompanied by a support person.

The manager must supply the clinician with a detailed description of the behaviour that has been deemed to be unhelpful or inadequate, and a statement outlining how the problem has come to light—through complaints, observations, and so on.

Negative aspects and outcomes of the behaviour in question must be explained. This should be done using specifics. General statements—such as 'our patients should not be upset' or 'nurses have to uphold the ethical principles of their profession'—are so vague as to be useless. It is best to start with the specific instances involved in the case at hand, and to broaden the relevant underlying principles to general cases later.

If the clinician agrees with the facts of the report, the manager can ask whether the clinician would act in the same way in future similar cases, or whether there might be other options. In this way the manager can identify possible attitudinal or knowledge deficits.

Steps in dealing with a major issue

This portion of the text explores the steps to be taken by a nurse manager in dealing with a major issue. These steps can be summarised as follows.

1. Adhere to the healthcare facility's formal procedure for dealing with major issues.
2. Meet with the nurse in private, and conduct the meeting with an assurance of confidentiality.
3. Supply the clinician with a detailed description of the behaviour that has been deemed to be unhelpful or inadequate, and a statement outlining how the problem has come to light—through complaints, observations, and so on.
4. Explain negative aspects and outcomes of the behaviour in question. This should be done using specific examples.
5. Ask whether the clinician would act in the same way in future similar cases—thus identifying possible attitudinal or knowledge deficits.
6. Provide the clinician with a specific plan of action—including measurable milestones and outcomes, and an indication of the help that can be provided by the organisation.
7. Arrange an agreed date to review progress towards satisfactory performance.

The next step in the process is to provide the clinician with a specific plan of action. This should include measurable milestones and outcomes, and an indication of the help that can be provided by the organisation. Such help might include in-house training, enrolment in relevant external courses, mentoring by other clinicians, or counselling.

The final step is to have an agreed date to review progress towards satisfactory performance. This needs to be realistic. On the one hand, the organisation expects satisfactory performance from its employees; on the other hand, the 'unhelpful' clinician might very well be angry at the situation. It is worth the effort and time to get the person 'on side' with the corrective program. An angry or resentful person makes for a poor learner! (Christie & Kleiner 2000).

Dealing with an angry nurse

The workplace seems, increasingly, to be developing into a stressful and angry place. Angry outbursts are almost an expected response to stressors—such as increasing workloads, loss of resources, and a lack of privacy (produced by open-plan workplaces, intrusive emails, and mobile phone messages). The rising tide of anger has been identified as a destroyer of team morale and a creator of anxiety—resulting in a hostile and underproductive work environment (Johnson & Indvik 2001).

The nurse manager should be mindful that anger can be caused by organisational factors as well as by personal factors. It is wrong to assume that the anger is a fixed personality trait that cannot be altered. Often the anger is an expression of stress caused by overwork (Johnson & Indvik 2001). The manager should be looking at other factors that might be modified to reduce stress—such as workload distribution, levels of client acuity, and rostering patterns.

> 'It is wrong to assume that the anger is a fixed personality trait that cannot be altered.'

If the problem is personally based, the following steps can be applied (Johnson & Indvik 2001).

- Meet with the clinician privately, and be prepared to suspend judgment until the facts of the case are established.
- Keep the clinician focused on the issue under consideration. It is quite common for an angry person to unleash a torrent of grievances. The manager must be firm in keeping the person on track; otherwise the possibility of an effective outcome is diminished.
- Validate the clinician's anger. Everyone gets angry at some time. The issue is not solely about the person's anger—it is also about the acceptable limits of anger, and what can be done about correcting the conditions that are causing the anger. Outline the consequences for the clinician and for the organisation if the angry behaviour continues.
- The manager should consider whether he or she is a cause of the clinician's anger. If so, is the manager an appropriate agent of mediation? Would it be better to withdraw and involve a neutral party?
- Allow for a cooling-off period. How badly is the anger affecting the clinician's performance? Is there an opportunity for reasonable adjustment?

Dealing with a bully

Bullying in the workplace can be defined as repeated, unreasonable, and inappropriate less-favourable treatment of one person by another (or others).

> 'Bullying is repeated, unreasonable, and inappropriate less-favourable treatment of one person by another.'

Bullying by colleagues and managers is a major cause of anxiety, stress, anger, distrust, and diminished work performance (Hannabuss 1998).

Bullying has been identified as a common form of indoctrinating new workers into the organisation and as a way of ensuring uniform behaviours by punishing individuals who do not conform to group norms. It is particularly endemic in hierarchically structured organisations—of which health care is an example (Archer 1999).

There is no evidence that people are 'born bullies'. Rather, bullying is a learned behaviour—which means that it should be capable of being 'unlearned' in many cases.

The method for dealing with allegations of bullying is the same as that set out above for major breaches of discipline and practice—with the proviso that the manager should be careful to keep focused on the bully, not the bully's victim.

The manager as bully

Managers have been identified as a major source of hostile and bullying behaviours (Field 1999). Although this behaviour is destructive in itself, it has greater implications for an organisation because managers who show that bullying is an 'effective' way of getting things done encourage bullying behaviours in subordinates (Archer 1999).

Bullying by managers can be quite subtle. The Box on page 91 lists some examples of bullying by managers.

Organisations must recognise that managers can be bullies, and should establish anti-bullying policies that (Work Cover Corporation 2000):

▶ clearly spell out unacceptable behaviours;
▶ establish appropriate lines of communication—for example, if a manager is the bully, the victim must be able to lodge a complaint with an officer who occupies a superior organisational position than the manager;
▶ establish quality assurance and workplace health-and-safety audit mechanisms that can uncover and track bullying behaviour; and
▶ react swiftly to reports of bullying.

Examples of bullying by managers

- disproportionate allocation of unpleasant duties;
- refusal of release for training;
- overreaction to trivial mistakes;
- withholding important information and resources, and reducing the availability of existing resources; and
- stealing the credit for others' ideas, and belittling the achievements of others.

Adapted from Collis (2001) and Jetson & Associates (2003)

Bullying must be seen as a serious breach of practice and organisational policy, and should be dealt with accordingly.

Conclusion

Unhelpful behaviours are a major concern for managers. Most of these behaviours can be dealt with at local level and handled by the manager who acts as counsellor and mentor. However, serious behaviours (such as bullying) require a formal process of identification and rectification.

The nurse manager must act ethically towards any clinician who is the subject of concern. The manager should maintain an open mind and be an objective investigator. Managers should not be swayed by bias or rely on heuristic devices to create a false air of certainty about the staff behavioural problems with which they deal.

Managers must never lose sight of the bigger organisational picture, and should be aware that this might be making a significant contribution to the behaviour of concern.

Managers should also be aware of the possibility that they might abuse their own positions of power. Such awareness, and the ability to respond appropriately to challenging or unhelpful staff behaviours, are generally not innate qualities. They must be fostered through organisa-tional policy and practices, and supported by appropriate training and human-management resources.

'Managers should also be aware of the possibility that they might abuse their own positions of power.'

Chapter 9

Managing Performance

Caroline Mulcahy

Introduction

Managing performance is a vital management skill if nurse managers are to inspire, motivate, and lead their teams to clinical excellence. Performance management includes the evaluation of an individual's work practice, the review of goals, the setting of new objectives, and career planning.

A variety of terms is used to describe performance management—including 'appraisal', 'performance appraisal', 'individual performance review' (IPR), and 'performance-improvement strategies'. Whichever term is used, the nurse manager should view performance management as offering a person a 'helping hand'. For the individual, it should be associated with a feeling of achievement and optimism about possibilities for the future.

It is not unusual to hear nurses say that they dread performance

> 'The nurse manager should view performance management as offering a person a "helping hand".'

management—whether it be a review of themselves or their conducting a review of others. Many performance reviews are not managed well because they focus on written goals and outcomes that are meaningless and are not followed up. In these instances, practical measures that address the 'why' and 'how' of doing something are not given sufficient consideration, and the exercise can become merely a process of generating paper. A thorough *individual* performance review is critical—and such an exercise is beneficial for both the nurse and the manager.

Effective performance management requires the nurse manager to be perceptive about individual employees if a performance plan is to be tailored to meet the needs of both manager and employee. Having agreed on a performance plan, the manager and the employee can then use this plan as an ongoing guide to their shared objectives and development needs.

Performance review (PR) discussions then enable assessment and review of performance against these objectives and needs, while also forming the basis for decisions on such matters as promotion, reclassification, training, educational needs, support needs and, in some circumstances, disciplinary action.

> 'Nurses must be nurtured and looked after if they are to remain on staff.'

Importance of performance management

The global shortage of nurses has heightened the challenge of recruiting *and* retaining qualified staff. Once they have been recruited, nurses must be nurtured and looked after if they are to remain on staff. In addition to individualised programs of orientation, mentoring, and preceptoring at the *beginning* of employment, an *ongoing* process of support—both personally and professionally—is required.

Staff satisfaction and staff performance are vital to patient satisfaction, and it is a manager's role to recognise when staff members are dissatisfied or when the performance of team members falls below an acceptable standard. Once aware of issues, the manager must respond in a timely, objective, unemotional, unbiased, and effective manner. Ignoring a problem and hoping that it might 'go away' is not a solution; problems will continue, often escalating until addressed.

Performance matters to both employees and managers. Most nurses go to work to contribute to the workplace. Once there, they want to feel valued and respected through acknowledgment and praise for a job well done. Performance management is thus a partnership that values staff. Done properly, it can empower staff members to make decisions, to accept responsibility for these decisions, and to be accountable.

In addition to being an evaluation of performance, PR should also be an opportunity for confidential discussions about the workplace in general; managers can learn much about their area of responsibility during such discussions. The Box below lists some of the features that make performance management important.

Importance of performance review

Performance review provides opportunities for nurse managers to:
- raise issues or concerns;
- reflect on practices and performance;
- acknowledge achievements;
- discuss training and development needs;
- promote activities; and
- plan careers.

PR is an opportunity for both the nurse and the nurse manager to clarify what is expected of the nurse, and to agree on priorities for improvement and development. Positive feedback, support, and recognition of achievement all enhance a person's ability to perform more effectively—but this must be based on a clear understanding of the actual role to be performed.

Positives and negatives of performance review

Performance management can be difficult. Many staff members view performance appraisal as a negative experience in which their performances are criticised, but in which solutions are absent and supports are inadequate. From the management perspective, many managers view the appraisal as being merely a time-consuming exercise. However, if conducted properly, performance reviews can be a positive experience. The Box on page 96 lists some of the positives and negatives of performance appraisal.

'If conducted properly, performance reviews can be a positive experience.'

Positives and negatives of performance appraisal

Positives

The positive aspects of performance review include:
- time to reflect on job;
- clarification of role and career pathway;
- 'quality time' with the manager and feedback from senior staff;
- identification of training needs;
- increased motivation;
- increased job satisfaction; and
- potential for better teamwork.

Negatives

The negative aspects of performance review include:
- the time-consuming nature of the review;
- the difficulties involved in conducting PR well;
- potential damage to relationships and trust;
- increased paperwork; and
- difficulty in measuring performance.

Role clarification

Clarifying a person's role in any given work area is the manager's responsibility. This clarification begins when a person considers applying for a job and requests a position description. The next opportunity to clarify and discuss role expectation is at the job interview, followed by a verbal offer and acceptance of the position. Following initial employment, managers should meet with the individual to discuss and explain his or her position description more thoroughly.

This early meeting is the key to role clarification and role expectation—and is the first step in effective performance management. During such a discussion, both parties can discuss the specific job to be performed, together with a wider discussion of the roles and contributions of other members of the team. Performance management is effective and measurable only when both the nurse and the manager have a clear understanding of the functioning of the whole team.

Conducting performance reviews
Frequency of reviews

Following employment, most contracts specify a probationary period—which usually includes an orientation program. At the completion of the program, there is an opportunity to ascertain whether the person has settled in, and to discuss any issues that have arisen with respect to the workplace and the expected performance.

After this initial discussion, a PR should occur whenever required or requested. To be effective, performance management should occur on an ongoing basis at a time when it is most relevant to reward good practice or to review sub-standard performance. Essentially this means that a person should be commended at the time that he or she is observed to have performed well. Conversely, when performance falls below what is expected, the most appropriate person should privately counsel the staff member as close to the incident as possible.

'Performance management should occur when it is most relevant to reward good practice or to review sub-standard performance.'

There should be an interim review at six months. After this, PR usually occurs on an annual basis. The Box below provides a recommended timeframe for individual performance review.

Timing of performance review

Initial
Appointment to position
Orientation
Preceptoring and/or mentoring

At 6 months
Discuss and appraise performance so far
Set and agree goals and learning needs in a performance plan

At 12 months
Individual performance review
Review and discuss performance against the above performance plan
- assessment and evaluation
- feedback and reward
- agree on supports and training requirements
Implement and monitor agreed performance plan

No longer than 12 months
Another individual performance review

Environment

The performance discussion should be conducted in a quiet place in a friendly, professional, and positive manner. Because most reviews usually occur annually, the nurse manager should allow a reasonable time for the review—perhaps 1–2 hours—so that the person under review feels relaxed, unhurried, respected, and valued. Particular attention should be given to body language and ensuring that no barriers are placed between the manager and the nurse. The Box below provides some tips on ensuring a suitable environment for a performance review.

Ensuring a suitable PR environment

To ensure a suitable environment for effective performance review, the nurse manager should:

- choose a quiet room, with no interruptions;
- turn off pagers;
- divert telephone calls;
- place a 'do not disturb' sign on the door;
- ensure that the conversation cannot be overheard; and
- dedicate time and attention to the process.

Who should perform a review?

Usually, a nurse manager conducts a performance review of his or her staff. However, this works well only with a small team. With a larger team, performance review should be delegated among the senior nursing staff members who have received appropriate training. In a large team, this means that no more than 15–20 nurses are accountable to any one person. With a larger number, the reviewer might have to rely on the perceptions of others, or mere hearsay. This can be inaccurate and judgmental. Limiting numbers means that more trusting relationships are developed, that communication is enhanced, and that the review involves ongoing constructive feedback with a view to personal development.

The reviewer and the nurse under review should work alongside one another on a regular basis before the performance review. The reviewer should be someone whom the nurse respects as a professional role model, counsellor, and teacher. As a 'coach', the reviewer can empower the nurse to grow and perform to his or her highest potential.

Preparation for a review

In preparation for the review, the nurse's job description (or position description) should be read thoroughly. This provides a description of the role and responsibilities of the nurse—including the required level of knowledge and clinical competence and the agreed reporting mechanisms.

A convenient meeting time and place should be arranged with the person. This should be done a couple of weeks before the meeting.

The manager should ensure that the nurse to be reviewed has the relevant paperwork. This includes the person's job or position description and any performance review form that is to be completed. If the current review is a repeat PR discussion, the manager should ensure that the person has a copy of the previous paperwork—which should include agreed goals and a performance plan for the previous period.

Before the meeting, the reviewer should gather as much information as possible by personally observing the individual while he or she is working. The appraiser should also review any feedback on the person—such as reports from preceptors, mentors, and multidisciplinary staff, comments from patients and their families, and observations from other visitors to the work area.

Before the appraisal, the nurse under review should assess his or her own performance by reflecting on previous objectives, performance, and practice. All results should be documented, including what has *not* been achieved.

Key points in performance review

- prepare and agree on a time and place;
- gather thoughts, information, evidence, and feedback;
- complete documentation before meeting;
- put the person at ease and ensure confidentiality;
- remain clear and objective;
- follow a plan or process;
- allow enough time;
- document the discussion and agreed outcomes; and
- sign the record and keep copies for further reviews.

Style of a review

The performance review process should be a 'purposeful conversation' (Ainsworth, Smith & Millership 2002). This can occur only if the person under review understands the reason for the review. The reviewer should therefore begin by explaining the purpose of the meeting, describing the process to be followed, and outlining the expected outcomes.

The reviewer should ensure that the discussion begins in a positive way by allowing the employee to lead the discussion by reviewing previous goals, achievements, and skill needs. In turn, the reviewer should give positive feedback by acknowledging and reaffirming these comments. Discussion should be encouraged by asking open-ended questions and asking the reviewee to detail certain experiences or situations.

The reviewer should ensure that the discussion is structured and time-limited. To facilitate this, a list of items can be used to guide the conversation, thus ensuring that all issues are discussed within the meeting time. The discussion should be focused on one topic at a time—which is discussed in full, and summarised. The reviewer should ensure that agreement is reached before moving on.

If previous goals have not been achieved, the reasons should be discussed—including the barriers or resource problems. An action plan should be formulated to address these difficulties.

Documentation should be exchanged, allowing time for both parties to read what the other has written. A future plan for the next appraisal period should be agreed upon. This should include training and development needs, new goals, key performance outcomes, and specific outcomes.

Skills required for performance review

Skills required to conduct a PR include the ability to:
- plan;
- provide constructive feedback;
- communicate effectively;
- listen actively;
- encourage, motivate, and reward; and
- assess, monitor, and evaluate performance objectively.

Documentation of reviews

Performance review should always be carefully documented. This provides a record for the reviewer and the person under review and allows progress to be assessed against a performance plan and expected outcomes.

In many performance reviews, forms are completed by the employee before the discussion takes place. This ensures that thought, planning, and reflection occur before the review. The person can also use this documentation as a guide during the discussion, thus facilitating the raising of issues and an organised review of performance.

The forms do not have to be complicated. Indeed, they are easier to use if they are short and easy to follow. Areas of performance that should be covered include:

▶ achievements during the previous 12-month period;
▶ individualised performance objectives or goals for the next 12 months;
▶ identification of areas for performance improvement (including an action plan, supports required; and a timeframe for the improvements to be achieved);
▶ discussion of the barriers to achieving the agreed objectives;
▶ areas for future growth and skill development (which might include an area of specific interest or a portfolio relevant to the ward area);
▶ outcomes of joint problem-solving (which includes identification and resolution of any problems related to the employee and performance); and
▶ any other comments or discussion points raised by either the manager or the nurse.

All PR forms should include the supports to be put in place to help the individual develop. Training requirements, support strategies, timelines, follow-up, and follow-through can all become important in a legal context. Proper documentation is therefore crucial.

To protect both parties in cases of disciplinary action or dismissal, an improvement plan (including strategies and supports) must have been clearly articulated and put into effect. Documentation of poor performance must have been provided to the person—thus making him or her aware of dissatisfaction, and providing an opportunity to improve performance.

'Documentation of poor performance must be provided—thus making the person aware of dissatisfaction, and providing an opportunity to improve performance.'

Supports

Supports include any inputs to improve a person's knowledge, skills, abilities, competencies, or confidence. They can include:

▶ counselling and coaching;
▶ on-the-job training;

▶ offering to move the person to a more suitable area of practice;
▶ provision of a preceptor or mentor;
▶ participation in broader activities (for example, case discussions, projects, research); and
▶ attendance at courses, seminars, in-service programs, or conferences.

Key performance indicators

Key performance indicators (KPIs) are individualised performance goals tailored to the person's position, role expectation, and personal development. To be effective, the person must take 'ownership' of his or her KPIs, must undertake to accomplish them within a certain time, and must agree upon the resources required to achieve them. In turn, the manager acknowledges the KPIs and undertakes to provide feedback to the person regarding progress in achieving them.

> 'The person must take "ownership" of his or her key performance indicators.'

Effective feedback

Feedback strategies are intended to improve and develop the person being reviewed.

Feedback should:
▶ be given at appropriate times;
▶ be specific, factual, and objective (rather than general, emotional, and subjective); and
▶ be supportive, non-judgmental, and outcome-based.

Feedback should *not*:
▶ be a one-way conversation led by the manager;
▶ be focused on a person's personality, character, or beliefs; or
▶ be judgmental, threatening, or intimidating.

In providing feedback during a review discussion, it is important that the manager remains focused and concentrates on specific occurrences as examples. A performance review is concerned with *performance*, not personality. It is easier to change a person's behaviour and work performance than it is to conduct a psychotherapy session. When giving either positive or negative feedback, nurse managers should therefore provide *real* examples of performance or anecdotes of *real* situations. If the nurse being reviewed attempts to appraise or criticise the manager, the conversation should be steered back to the purpose of the discussion.

Conducting difficult performance reviews

In conducting effective performance reviews in difficult situations, nurse managers should:
- listen to any perceived problems;
- provide helpful feedback and guidance;
- avoid conflict and disputes;
- provide support to address learning needs and skill acquisition;
- reward, coach, and support staff;
- discuss career expectations;
- empower staff to suggest solutions and innovations; and
- provide opportunities for second opinions or referral to human-resource personnel.

Poor performance and disagreements

However difficult it might be to address a certain issue, disagreements and problems should not be ignored. Nurse managers should organise a time to meet with the person, and begin the review process again.

When addressing such issues, nurse managers should:
▶ be honest about the problem, discuss it fairly, and listen to what the nurse has to say;
▶ review the original performance plan to ensure that it was clear, understood, realistic, and achievable;
▶ discuss the position and role again, paying particular attention to role clarity;
▶ set and agree on a new plan—with a short timeframe for further discussion; and
▶ follow up on the agreed plan.

A learning contract can be presented in the form of a written document that specifies problems to be addressed and the strategies agreed by all parties. This ensures that corrective measures are actually put in place. If possible, education staff should be involved in the writing of learning contracts (and any associated KPIs).

In managing these difficult issues, the manager should ensure that he or she is aware of body language and inappropriate reactions. If it appears that a conflict is likely to arise, the manager should stop the conversation. There should be no expressions

'If it appears that a conflict is likely to arise, the manager should stop the conversation. There should be no expressions of anger.'

of anger. Rather, an understanding and supportive manner is required at all times.

If, despite the best efforts of the manager, a dispute remains about the outcome of the PR, either person can seek the second opinion of a more senior nurse or referral to the organisation's human-resources department. Most organisations have comprehensive policies and procedures in place that explain how to deal with grievances—including the process for appeals and access to coaching and counselling.

Conclusion

The purpose of individual performance reviews is to develop staff members in undertaking specific jobs, to broaden their skills, and to help them to grow and reach their full potentials. Nurse managers are responsible for providing direction, assistance, and supports, and staff members are responsible for utilising their reviews to advance their career development.

Staff members need to understand what is expected of them in their various roles, and want to feel valued in those roles. Effective communication among all members of a team facilitates improved performance, increases satisfaction, and leads to improved quality of care.

Undertaking a process of PR demonstrates an interest and commitment to the development and professional growth of the team. If the whole organisation undertakes this, a learning organisation develops. In such an organisation, a culture of ongoing reflection and learning permeates all levels—thus promoting optimal utilisation of all available resources.

'In a learning organisation, a culture of ongoing reflection and learning permeates all levels.'

Chapter 10

Managing Risk

Therese Caine and Cathie Steele

Introduction

> It is simply not acceptable for patients to be harmed by the same health
> care system that is supposed to offer healing and comfort.

KOHN, CORRIGAN & DONALDSON (1999)

Risk management is a relatively new concept in health care. Nurses have always
prided themselves on doing the best for patients, and the idea that patients could
be harmed by nursing care is alien. As organisational decentralisation has
occurred, the responsibilities of middle managers have increased. Nurse
managers have taken responsibility for management of the continuum of care,
of people, and of budgets. Responsible management in these areas includes
managing the associated risks.

A key characteristic of an effective manager is managing risks proactively—
rather than reacting when things go wrong. Managing risks proactively is about
making an assessment of what can possibly go wrong, developing a plan to

manage these risks, acting on the plan, harnessing the efforts of the team, and then recognising the improvements.

Consumers as drivers of change

Consumers of health care are driving change and want to know that health professionals will keep them safe. However, if an adverse event occurs, consumers want to know that all will be done to prevent it happening again, that an apology will be made, and that clinicians will speak to them and involve them in the solution (Vincent, Young & Phillips 1994). As an advocate for the consumer, the nurse manager oversees the overall picture of patient care and is accountable for coordinating nurses and other health professionals to deliver the best and least risky care possible.

> 'Consumers of health care are driving change and want to know that health professionals will keep them safe.'

Why things go wrong

Preventing errors and improving safety for patients requires a systems approach in order to modify the conditions that contribute to errors. People working in health care are among the most educated and dedicated workforce in any industry. The problem is not bad people; the problem is that the system needs to be made safer.

KOHN, CORRIGAN & DONALDSON (1999)

Research on learning from failures in health care is relatively sparse. However, evidence from other industries reveals a rich seam of knowledge about the nature of failure that is relevant to health care.

Nurses are highly motivated and committed to doing the best-possible job and to doing no harm. Patient safety is a concept that seems so simple and fundamental to clinical practice that it is actually difficult to get some nurses to recognise that patients are often harmed by the system and by care interventions.

> 'It is actually difficult to get some nurses to recognise that patients are often harmed by the system and by care interventions.'

The Box below lists some conditions that have been associated with adverse events:

Conditions associated with adverse events

The following conditions have been found to be associated with adverse events:
- diffuse responsibility (due to the fact that many people and departments are frequently involved in the care of any given patient);
- poor communication and teamwork;
- professional 'silos' with rigid hierarchies;
- intolerance to criticism;
- time pressure and high workload;
- unmotivated staff;
- deficient leadership and management;
- little education on education and research;
- a focus on targets and goals that are not related to the quality of care;
- technically complex tasks; and
- a lack of appropriate policies and procedures being used to guide care.

Adapted from Reason (1997) and Donaldson & Muir Gray (1998)

Some of the factors listed in the Box are usually present in all organisations. There is a strong consensus that the intrinsic culture of health care places too much emphasis on human error rather than on designing systems that incorporate safeguards against error (Berwick 1989; Leape 1994). Blaming individuals for mistakes results in requiring people to try harder, or be more careful.

It is appropriate that individuals in health care must be held to account for their actions—in particular if there is evidence of gross negligence or recklessness, or of criminal behaviour. However, in the great majority of cases, the causes of serious failures stretch far beyond the actions of the individuals immediately involved. Safety is dynamic; it is not a static situation.

'Safety is dynamic; it is not a static situation.'

In a socially and technically complex field such as health care, a huge number of factors is at work to influence the likelihood of failure. The Box on page 108 describes two elements that have been identified in failure analysis.

Active failures and latent conditions

Two elements that have been identified in failure analysis are:
- *active failures:* 'unsafe acts' committed by those working at the 'sharp end' of a system; these are usually short-lived and are often unpredictable; and
- *latent conditions:* conditions that can develop over time and lie dormant before combining with other factors or active failures to breach a system's safety defences; these are long-lived and can be identified and removed before they cause an adverse event.

Adapted from Reason (1997)

Within nursing, much research has focused on identifying those patient outcomes that can be directly linked to nursing interventions and considering the nature of errors made in nursing practice (Meurier 2000; Benner et al. 2002). Certain adverse patient outcomes have been identified as being more closely linked with nursing interventions. These include:
- medication administration errors;
- patient falls;
- pressure wounds;
- nosocomial infections; and
- unplanned readmissions to hospital.

In addition to these patient outcomes, a range of contributing nursing work factors—including lack of attentiveness and judgment, and poor advocacy and intervention on behalf of patients—has been identified (Benner et al. 2002). Nurse staffing issues—such as competency and skill mix—can also affect patient outcomes (Aiken et al. 2002; Needleman et al. 2002).

Human error can sometimes be the factor that immediately precipitates a serious failure, but there are usually deeper systemic factors at work. If these are addressed, this will prevent the error or mitigate its consequences.

'Human error can immediately precipitate a serious failure, but there are usually deeper systemic factors at work.'

The aim of all improvements is to make systems safer. This involves looking to improve the systems of health care, reducing reliance on human memory, ensuring safe working hours, improving ability to work together in teams (rather than as individuals), and simplifying and standardising work practices wherever possible.

The international perspective

Retrospective studies that assess adverse events occurring to patients in acute care have been the catalysts for an increased focus on safety by the public, the media, and the healthcare system itself. In addition major investigations have been undertaken into systemic failures in health services around the world (Vecchi 2003). Although hospital services differ from one another in various ways, there are similarities in the findings of these studies. In particular, health services need to have in place (Vecchi 2003):

▶ systems to support safe practice on the part of those who work in the health system;
▶ effective credentialling and performance-management systems;
▶ improved data and information for safer care;
▶ increased involvement of consumers in improving healthcare safety;
▶ redesigned systems of health care to facilitate a culture of safety;
▶ a much improved awareness and understanding of healthcare safety by all stakeholders.

Following on from these studies and inquiries, governments of major Western healthcare services have set up organisations to drive improvements in patient safety and quality. In some countries legislation has been passed to define the statutory duty of quality required of healthcare organisations, and failure to meet such standards can result in withdrawal of accreditation as a health service.

The nature of risk management

Risk management is an integral component of good management practice. The 'Risk Management Standard' (Standards Australia 1999) offers a systematic framework for undertaking a cycle of quality improvement and problem-solving. This formal step-by-step process, which can be applied to all elements within a work environment, involves five steps. These are summarised in the Box below.

Five steps in risk management

The five steps in risk management recommended by Standards Australia (1999) are:
• establishing the context for risk management;
• risk-identification;
• risk-analysis;
• risk-evaluation and treatment; and
• ongoing processes for monitoring and review.

Categories of risk within an area include:

▶ patient care-related risks (infection, pressure wounds, falls, medications);
▶ clinical staff risks (staff competence, credentialling, discipline);
▶ employee risks (occupational injury, work environment);
▶ property risks (fire, equipment damage, patient valuables);
▶ financial risks (staff overtime, investment in equipment); and
▶ ward or service governance risks (communication, effective management, compliance with policies and procedures, change management, selling the message of the governing body, and so on).

Establishing a risk-management system

To ensure a safer workplace it is important to have an understanding of:

▶ the identification of risk;
▶ the analysis of risk;
▶ the prioritisation of risk; and
▶ the management of risk.

Each of these is discussed below.

Identification of risks

Risks can be identified retrospectively or prospectively. If possible, risks should be identified from existing information such as:

▶ incidents or near misses reported by staff, patients, or family members;
▶ evaluation of current or proposed work processes;
▶ complaints;
▶ patient satisfaction surveys;
▶ medical record reviews; and
▶ clinical audits.

Establishing a risk-management system

To ensure a safer workplace it is important to have an understanding of:

• the identification of risk;
• the analysis of risk;
• the prioritisation of risk; and
• the management of risk.

These matters are discussed in greater detail in this section of the text.

Analysis of risks

The two factors to be considered when analysing risk are: (i) the *likelihood* or *probability* of the event happening; and (ii) the *consequences* or *severity* of that event. The first of these (probability) can be assessed along a continuum from *remote* to *frequent*, whereas the second (severity) can rate from *catastrophic* to *minor*. In many cases, these assessments are qualitative and involve the best educated guess.

When assessing a risk, consideration is given to actual events and potential events—including an assessment of 'close calls'. In this way, there is both a proactive and a reactive risk management response adapted to suit any facility.

It is a good idea to ensure that a high-level decision-making group in the organisation is involved in analysing risks and establishing the risk-management framework.

Prioritisation of risk

If numbers are allocated to the *severity and probability* categories for either an actual event or a potential event, a score can be obtained. Events can then be ranked. These rankings can then be used for comparative analysis and for prioritising the event. Risk-rating can also help in the prioritisation of risks associated with proposed new treatments or services.

Management of risk

Managing or treating the risks requires taking action to improve the situation. The process for developing an action plan includes the following:

- utilising a team approach to develop the plan;
- prioritising the risks according to level of impact and likelihood;
- assessing the cause using the literature on the subject and professional judgment; this involves using a cause-and-effect process (see Chapter 12, page 135) to clarify team deliberations and to identify root causes of the identified risk;
- prioritising the most likely and most serious contributing factors;
- identifying a range of effective strategies to reduce the risk;
- agreeing on: (a) who will take responsibility for managing the strategy implementation; (b) the timeframe for implementation; and (c) how improvement will be measured; and
- agreeing on a monitoring and communication process.

Monitoring and evaluating improvements

Once an improvement action is in place, it is necessary to collect data in relation to the improvement and to review these data within the team. In addition, other services in the health service should be informed of the nature and progress of improvements.

An internal benchmarking exercise involving teams within the organisation might be established, or an external benchmarking exercise might be organised involving another organisation that is making a particular improvement. Whichever pathway is chosen, improvements will accrue though ongoing learning and sharing of information.

Caring for patients harmed by treatment

If a serious adverse event happens patients, relatives, and staff members can all be traumatised. If such a situation is handled in an insensitive or inadequate manner, this will compound the situation. In contrast, if there is immediate, open, and honest discussion of the event, the impact can be limited.

'If there is immediate, open, and honest discussion of the event, the impact can be limited.'

Patients can have powerful reactions to such an adverse event. They feel let down by the people in whom they placed their trust. Moreover, they usually require further care in the same system, and often by the same people who were involved in the adverse event (Vincent 2001). If the nurse manager is sensitive and skilled in dealing with these events, there will be reduced anger, improved safety, better communication, increased satisfaction, and, possibly, reduced litigation.

Supporting staff involved in serious incidents

The consequences of an error in health care can be catastrophic for a patient, and it is not uncommon for an error to be seen as 'unacceptable'. When an individual nurse perceives error as being 'unacceptable', that person is more likely to perceive any performance that is below the accepted level of excellence as constituting *personal failure* (Hewett 2001). This leads to significant personal and professional conflict.

There are usually many factors that lead to adverse events. These factors can be personal or systemic. The problem for the nurse manager is how best to support staff members who are involved in adverse events. The aim should be to reduce the trauma of the event and to assist the individual nurses to contribute to the learning of the organisation. To do this, a culture of openness and honesty must exist—a culture in which individuals are supported, and in which the organisation demonstrates that it can learn from such events.

'A culture of openness and honesty . . . in which individuals are supported, and in which the organisation demonstrates that it can learn from events.'

Dealing with clinical complaints

A complaint about a service might come from a patient, carers, or staff members. It is important that complaints are heard according to a timely process and that the complaint is acknowledged and dealt with in a private and confidential manner.

Every attempt should be made to hear the complainant and to resolve the issue in a positive way. If this is done, many complaints can be resolved without their escalating out of proportion. When it is impossible to resolve a complaint at the point of care, the nurse manager should seek assistance from the complaints manager, quality manager, or patient liaison officer.

Root cause analysis

When significant and harmful events occur, it is important that the event is reported and managed well. This includes managing the immediate situation for the patient and family, supporting the staff members (who are frequently traumatised), and ensuring that appropriate investigations are put into place to determine the underlying systemic factors. Many hospitals today have clinical risk managers who will assist in notification of insurers, investigation of the incident, and follow-up to improve the hospital processes.

In any significant event, a root cause analysis should be carried out as part of a philosophy of building a *culture of safety* rather than a *culture of blame*. The goal of root cause analysis is to find out

▶ what happened;
▶ why it happened; and
▶ what should be done to prevent its happening again.

In root cause analysis, basic and contributing causes are discovered. The goal, at all times, is to prevent a recurrence of the event.

The Box below summarises the key characteristics of root cause analysis.

Root cause analysis

The key characteristics of root cause analysis can be summarised as follows. Root cause analysis is:

- *inter-disciplinary*—involving those who are the most familiar with the situation and experts from various frontline services;
- *multi-level*—continually digging deeper at each level of cause and effect and asking the question: 'Why?';
- *systemic*—seeking to identify changes that need to be made to *systems*; and
- *impartial*—striving to be fair and balanced at every stage of the process.

Documentation and record-keeping

Nurses often consider themselves to be workers first and writers second (Richmond 2001). Documentation written by nurses is often criticised for lacking professional technique and containing redundant information, and this does appear to be the case when a patient's record is searched for evidence of what happened in relation to a particular event. It is often difficult to tell what happened and when.

It is important that nurses change negative views of documentation to ensure that it goes beyond merely recording the tasks performed. Documentation is evidence that demonstrates accountability. It identifies that care processes have been undertaken as planned, and that outcomes have been achieved. Evidence in the patient record also enables review of the care processes, identification of unplanned events and variances, and identification of needed improvements.

Coroners use the patient record as principal evidence when investigating the death of a patient. As health professionals, nurses have an obligation to ensure that the record—in the form of care pathways, daily charts, or progress notes—accurately reflects the events that occurred.

Statutory immunity

Health professionals want to provide the best possible care for patients and carers, and patients and carers have an expectation that those healthcare professionals (and the system in which they work) will provide safe high-quality care.

In many countries, the concepts of 'qualified privilege' and 'statutory immunity' are incorporated in legislation. These concepts encourage health professionals to participate in quality-improvement activities by providing for:

▶ the confidentiality of some documents and proceedings of healthcare quality committees or activities;

▶ protection of those documents and proceedings from being used in legal actions; and

▶ protection from legal liability for present and former members of healthcare quality committees who were acting in good faith in carrying out their responsibilities.

Such legislation seeks to achieve a balance between competing public interests—(i) the public interest in encouraging healthcare professionals to take part in quality assurance and improvement activities; and (ii) the public interest in having access to information about those activities.

Conclusion

Managing risk is an overarching aspect of the nurse manager's role. In providing clinical services, the nurse manager's paramount concern must be to en-sure the health and safety of patients and staff.

In establishing and maintaining a framework of risk management, improvements in patient safety should focus on:

> 'The nurse manager's paramount concern must be to ensure the health and safety of patients and staff.'

▶ establishing a culture of safety;

▶ implementing clinical and nursing practice improvements based on evidence and best practice;

▶ undertaking effective and open communication with patients;

▶ ensuring that care interventions are timely and that delays are minimised;

▶ 'working smarter' by changing mental models of what is possible in nursing practice;

▶ providing care that is equitable to all;

▶ sharing improvement successes with others; and

▶ maintaining a change momentum to ensure improvements are ongoing.

Chapter 11

Occupational Health and Safety

Janis Jansz

Introduction

The nature of nursing means that, throughout the world every day, many nurses are injured or become ill as a result of work. Causes include physical violence, ergonomic hazards (such as manual handling), exposure to infectious diseases (airborne, bloodborne, and direct contact), fatigue (due to physically and mentally demanding work), work organisation and shift work, radiation (ionising and non-ionising), handling toxic drugs, and exposure to chemicals.

Nurses are rarely taught about occupational health and safety (OHS). Nursing is a profession that is focused on providing the best possible care to patients within the restrictions of the resources provided. To deliver this care, nurses are sometimes pushed beyond their physical and mental limits, particularly when working an early shift after working a late shift on the previous day.

Nurse managers, whether employed by government departments or private organisations, are dependent on the work conditions and resources provided by that employer. They must therefore be advocates for their own occupational safety and health, and must be proactive in providing a high standard of OHS for the people in their area of responsibility.

Legal requirements

In most countries there is a legal requirement to provide sound occupational safety and health. Because requirements differ among jurisdictions, it is important for nurse managers to be familiar with the legal parameters of their particular workplaces.

There are two main types of OHS legislation. The first is a prescriptive statement of the minimum standards that must be met by employers and employees in order to provide a safe and healthy workplace. This type of law, which applies in the United States of America (USA), requires constant updating. The other type of legislation follows the Robens' (1972) philosophy of the United Kingdom (UK) and involves a duty of care on the part of all in the workplace. In both cases there is provision for fines if legal requirements are not met and if work-related hazards are not controlled. In some countries (for example, UK, Australia, and USA), a person can be imprisoned should death result from that person's actions or omissions in the workplace.

Hazards and risks

A *hazard* is anything that might result in: (i) death or injury to a person; (ii) harm to health; (iii) damage to property, equipment, or process; or (iv) loss to an organisation or individual. There are eight major groups of work-related hazards:

▶ physical (air quality, noise, electrical, heat, cold, radiation);
▶ chemical (solids, liquids, gases);
▶ ergonomic (manual handling, work equipment design, task design);
▶ mechanical (machinery);
▶ psychological (shift work, workload, bullying);
▶ biological (viral or bacterial infection);
▶ environmental (storms, earthquakes, terrorism); and
▶ general (slips, trips, falls).

Risk is defined as the likelihood of harmful human or property contact with the hazard. Risk assessment analyses the probability and consequences of contact with the hazard. The combination of probability and consequences of occurrence determines the degree of risk present.

Effective safety management includes consideration of everything that could go wrong including: (i) the design of the service; (ii) the working life of the people, premises, equipment, and products used; (iii) all work processes; (iv) the effects that the service might have on customers and the community; (v) the effects that the government and members of the community might have on the nurses; and (vi) the effects of the decommissioning of the organisation. Once the risk of any hazard causing harm has been established, risk-control strategies need to be implemented.

Risk control is as much about improving cost-effective management, as it is about avoiding or preventing losses. A 'no individual blame' system should be promoted so that people will not be afraid to report problems. Thus nurse managers need to encourage all staff members to report any workplace problems, so that the risk of the hazard causing harm can be eliminated, and OHS improved.

> 'A 'no individual blame' system should be promoted so that people will not be afraid to report problems.'

Something as simple as removing a trip hazard might prevent injury and the associated costs that result from providing health care for the injured person and investigating the accident. Repair or replacement costs can result from damage to equipment or work premises. If the injured person is a staff member, costs might include wages during absence from work, the loss of skill and experience, the cost of replacing the person until he or she is able to return to work, obtaining and training the replacement, and the potential lower work output of the replacement. Even if the employee is not able to work as efficiently as before the accident, full wages might still be necessary. There can also be other costs—such as decreased employee morale, increased labour conflict, and adverse media publicity. It is far more economical to spend money on safe work premises, practices, and employee actions than to spend money on the consequences of not having these preventive measures in place.

When providing a high standard of occupational safety and health, the nurse manager needs to consider seven main areas:

◗ work environment;
◗ products and equipment used;
◗ management factors (including work organisation);
◗ employees;
◗ contractors;

▶ patients and visitors; and

▶ community and legal requirements and expectations.

These can be developed as a simple model for safety management (see Figure 11.1, below). As can be seen in the model, risk control can be considered under the headings of: (i) inputs; (ii) work activities; and (iii) outputs. Each of these is considered below.

Areas → **Risk Control** → **Effective health and safety management**

▶ work environment
▶ products and equipment used
▶ management (including work organisation)
▶ employees
▶ contractors
▶ clients and visitors
▶ community/legal requirements and expectations

▶ for inputs
▶ for work activities
▶ for outputs

Figure 11.1 A model for occupational health and safety management
Author's presentation

Safety management for inputs

The first stage of the required program of hazard identification, assessment, and risk control is to minimise or eliminate hazards and risks of harm. This involves consideration of physical resources, human resources, and information (as illustrated in Figure 11.2, below). Each of these is discussed below in two typical settings in which nurse managers might find themselves responsible—in the context of a hospital setting and in a nursing agency.

Resources

▶ physical resources
▶ human resources ⟶ **Safety management inputs**
▶ information

Figure 11.2 A model for safety management inputs
Author's presentation

In a hospital
Physical resources

In a hospital setting, the *physical resources* that need to be considered are the design, selection, and construction of the workplace. The premises should be located in a safe area, built to meet service requirements, and constructed safely. Risk-control strategies must be considered in the design, selection, purchase, and installation of all equipment and products—which should be the safest and most efficient available. Employees who will use equipment (for example, a lifting hoist) or product (for example, hand-washing soap) should be involved in making decisions about the equipment or product purchased. This ensures the practicality of purchases and encourages a commitment to using the equipment or product safely.

Equipment should be designed to minimise the potential for human error. There should be sufficient equipment and products to perform the required tasks safely. Products should be available locally and should be available from more than one supplier. At least three days' supply of all consumables should be kept on the premises.

Equipment should have easily available parts from local suppliers and should be maintained by local contractors if possible. If components have to be sent from overseas, this can result in expensive delays. Suppliers should be partners in risk-control activities and have ongoing contracts with the organisation to promote commitment to high standards. Contractors' equipment and substances should also be considered in risk control because many core business activities, such as catering or cleaning, might be contracted out.

Human resources

In a hospital, the *human resources* that managers need to consider are recruitment and selection. The nurses who are selected should have a positive attitude to safety and be motivated to work safely. Nurse managers are leaders who have responsibility for planning, leading, and controlling work, and they therefore need to have a high level of knowledge about OHS, and be prepared to take responsibility for it.

'Nurses should have a positive attitude to safety and be motivated to work safely.'

Information

With regard to *information* in a hospital setting, consideration should be given to legislation, standards, codes of practice, guidance notes, organisational best practice, and any other technical and management information that relates to OHS.

In a nursing agency

To take another example, the same three safety-management inputs (physical resources, human resources, and information) can be considered in the setting of a nursing agency.

Physical resources

In this setting, the *physical resources* involved are similar to those of the hospital—the premises, products, and equipment used. However, an agency has additional responsibilities in that it sends its employees to many workplaces that are under the control of other employers. The agency manager should therefore check the premises, equipment, and products used at each location. Although the owner/occupier of the premises has a legal responsibility for safety, the agency also needs to ensure that its employees have a safe workplace, products, and equipment. Employees should not be sent to workplaces where the risk of hazards is not controlled.

Human resources

Obligations for *human resources* in a nursing agency are similar to those of a hospital, but agency nurses can be required to have an even wider variety of skills and safety knowledge than nurses who are based in a hospital. Agency nurses must constantly adapt to new premises, equipment, products, people, routines, and workplaces. When selecting nurses, an agency should select employees who are adaptable, and who are comfortable when asking for information. Ergonomically, if physical and mental health is to be maintained, it is important to have a person who fits a workplace, as well as ensuring that the workplace suits the nurse.

Information

Requirements for *information* in a nursing agency are also similar to those of a hospital. However, an agency has additional requirements because the nurse manager needs to provide information about new work-related situations. The agency must therefore constantly obtain information and communicate this information before the employee begins work. The agency can also use health-care organisations to provide orientation and OHS information for staff. It is also useful for the nurse manager to send agency nurses to the same workplace whenever possible—thus optimising familiarity with processes. An efficient way to check the occupational safety of any organisation is to ask for the safety management plan of that organisation, and to check its adequacy—complementing this with verbal reports from the nurses working there.

Safety management for work activities

As illustrated in Figure 11.1 (page 120), the second aspect of risk control is safety management for work activities. The objective of this part of the occupational program is to minimise or eliminate risks within business processes. Risk-control activities need to include: (i) the work environment; (ii) equipment and substances used; (iii) procedures; (iv) people; and (v) management systems. Each of these is discussed below.

Physical work environment

Factors that need to be considered in the *physical work environment* include the work premises, buildings, grounds, entrances and exits, and community areas that employees might reasonably be expected to use.

Equipment and products

When considering *equipment* and *products* used, risk control should include any hazards that can occur when equipment or products are used, handled, transported, or stored. Elimination of a hazard by purchasing the safest product possible maximises occupational safety and employee health.

All equipment must have regular maintenance and evaluation to ensure correct functioning. There should always be backup for equipment so that if one piece of equipment fails, another takes over. A policy that ensures equipment is replaced before wearing out should be instituted.

Safe work procedures

Hazard identification, risk assessment, and risk control must be included in the design stage of all *work procedures*. This includes an analysis of work and job safety that considers the location of the work, how each job will be done, the steps to be included, hazards that might occur when performing the job, preventive action to be taken to eliminate or minimise the risks of any hazards, standard of work required, and any certificates of competency required. When including safety management in the plan of work, the nurse manager should consider who will do the work, how many people will do it, the skills required to do it, the training and instruction required, the level of supervision needed, and how long each task should take.

> 'Hazard identification, risk assessment, and risk control must be included in the design stage of all work procedures.'

When implementing risk control into work procedures, the nurse manager should consider ways to eliminate particular hazards. Employees might be immunised against communicable diseases, or consideration might be given to ways of minimising the effects of hazards that cannot be controlled (for example, stress due to having to deal with multiple casualty events). As well as having an effective debriefing and support system, the organisation should be able to commence rehabilitation as soon as possible after any adverse health effect occurs.

With all procedures it is important to plan to be safe. Safe behaviour should be expected—and it should be rewarded by management. The promotion and practice of safe behaviour costs less than dealing with the consequences of accidents.

Safety management system

The risk-control program must include a *safety-management system* for each type of work. This should include the following:

▶ skilled supervision;

▶ consultation and cooperation;

▶ communication;

▶ competence;

▶ implementing work procedures;

▶ measuring, reviewing, and auditing performance;

▶ people; and

▶ security.

Each of these is considered below.

In providing *skilled supervision*, a nurse manager should set a personal example in promoting health and safety for all concerned. Safe procedures should be implemented after appropriate education has been provided. The nurse manager is then required to monitor performance and effectiveness.

In providing *consultation and cooperation*, the nurse manager needs to be team orientated in working with employees to develop and update practice, and in ensuring acceptance and effective implementation of such practice. All staff members must work together to decide how any deficiencies will be reported and rectified. It is important for the nurse manager to be involved in these activities because management has control of the resources and provides direction for work processes. It is important for the staff to be involved because they are the people most likely to identify any hazard risks or inefficiencies in procedures.

Consensus is required on what *communication* is necessary, what documentation should be involved, and how it can be designed to be clear, effective, and easy to use. Staff members must be trained to document carefully and accurately–because documentation might be called upon at any legal proceedings arising from an adverse incident. Important documentation should be stored in more than one form (for example, hardcopy and electronic)—to ensure that if one type of record is lost, another exists. An effective risk-reporting system needs to be implemented to facilitate any follow-up action that is required to control identified risks.

With respect to *competence*, the nurse manager must ensure that the training, qualifications, skills, and level of competence of nurses, and those who monitor them, are adequate to perform tasks to the required standard.

In *implementing work procedures*, the first-line supervisor is a critical person. The organisation needs to ensure that it has adequate systems in place to enable line managers to provide competent supervision and to manage work safely. The nurse manager must provide adequate human and material resources to

> 'It is important that employees are provided with enough time to work safely . ... many accidents happen when not enough time is allocated.'

ensure that the work is performed to the required standard. It is particularly important that employees are provided with enough time to work safely and that there are enough employees to do the work. Many accidents happen when not enough time is allocated.

A most important part of the safety-management system is *measuring, reviewing,* and *auditing performance*—and making changes as required. This can be achieved by having periodic inspections of work, documentation, and staff discussions, and by having outside consultants to evaluate performance.

When eliminating and minimising risks, one of the most important elements to consider are the *people* doing the work. This includes the effective placement of nurses, their competence for the job, and any health surveillance needed. Nurses must be encouraged to develop a culture in which they care for each other, as well as for their patients. This involves:

> 'Nurse managers should let their staff members know that they are valued.'

(i) working together as a team; (ii) performing work-related tasks to the required standard; (iii) being empowered; (iv) being consulted (and participating) in planning, implementing, and evaluating services and change; (v) having security of employment; and

(vi) communicating effectively. Nurse managers should let their staff members know that they are valued. Job security encourages employee commitment to the organisation and to occupational safety and health practices.

Bullying is an important hazard. This can be defined as any activity that 'harms, intimidates, threatens, victimises, undermines, offends, degrades or humiliates an employee' (WorkSafe WA 2003b, p. 1). Bullying can be perpetrated by a co-worker, a patient, or a visitor, and can cause stress leading to a stress-related illness, anxiety, sleep disturbances, fatigue, or depression. In severe cases, the person being bullied might even commit suicide. The hazard of bullying can be overcome by implementing anti-bullying strategies (see WorkSafe WA 2003b).

Many health-care organisations are so busy providing external 'customer care' that they forget to care for the health of their employees. Employee health promotion should become a corporate value for the organisation, and nurse managers should actively show care for the personal health of employees. For

> 'Nurse managers should actively show care for the personal health of employees.'

example, if employees complain of being tired at work, organisation (hours of work and patient allocation) can be examined and improved. Provision of education about personal factors should also be part of such a health-promotion program.

With regard to *security*, nurse managers should be aware that nurses are increasingly exposed to violence. Potential hazards should be eliminated by removing the cause of violence, and by replacing work processes that cause violence with less hazardous tasks. Solutions for overcoming these hazards should be tried—such as installing security systems, lighting work areas, setting up appropriate barriers, and reorganising work (such as by using job rotation for stressful situations). Training for how to deal with aggression and the provision of personal protective equipment is also desirable. Codes of practice for preventing and dealing with workplace violence are available (for example, WorkSafe WA 2003a).

Safety management of outputs

Output risk control is necessary to minimise risk arising from nurses' work activities, services provided, or information given. Any complaints from patients, members of the public, government organisations, or businesses must be investigated. Appropriate risk-control measures must be implemented, and steps should be taken to minimise any environmental pollution or damage. Most hospitals have waste-management procedures that minimise the amount of waste generated and that dispose of waste products according to legal guidelines. Employees should be supported when an investigation of an adverse event takes place. Work process and organisational causes must be considered.

The benefits

A sound occupational safety-management program results in:

- fewer human, material, and system losses;
- maximisation of business continuity through contingency plans for people, equipment, and products;
- optimum allocation of resources;
- a culture of controlling risks and promoting work-related safety;
- better managerial strategic decisions regarding business risks;
- good ideas, information, and resources across work groups promoting OHS;
- reduction in lost time through injury or disease;
- reduction in workers' compensation premiums;
- delivery of competitive advantage through cost-effective service;
- increased credibility of service;
- positive publicity and enhanced reputation; and
- increased likelihood of accreditation and recognition by relevant authorities.

Conclusion

An OHS management program is essential to the control and reduction of risk in nursing management. It provides public credibility for risk-management decisions, offers cost-effective service to the community, meets legal occupational safety and health requirements, and continuously improves business activities.

Chapter 12

Maximising the Quality Factor

Therese Caine and Cathie Steele

Introduction

Quality in health care has been defined as 'doing the right thing, the first time, in the right way, and at the right time' (NSW Health 2002). Consumers of health care expect that the services provided will be safe, effective, appropriate, consumer-focused, accessible, and efficient. The challenge for providers of health care is to monitor and improve systems continuously to satisfy these expectations.

Advances in scientific understanding, therapeutics, and technology in recent decades have resulted in better care, but these improvements have also introduced higher levels of complexity into systems without a companion system of evaluation—a system of evaluation that ensures the best possible care for patients. In

> 'Quality in health care is doing the right thing, the first time, in the right way, and at the right time.'

addition, the complexity of modern health care has increased the opportunities for system failures and human error. The concerns expressed by clinicians, consumers, governments, and the media have resulted in an increasing focus on quality and safety in Western healthcare systems over recent years.

The nurse manager is the pivotal person to lead the way in improving services within his or her area of responsibility. The establishment of standards of professional nursing practice, and the maintenance and evaluation of these standards, are central to the role of manager. As a professional, the nurse manager is required to be accountable for the quality of nursing services in his or her area of responsibility. This involves ensuring effective staff management, accountability of shift leaders after hours, relationship management with other members of the healthcare team, financial management, client and staff satisfaction, and service planning and implementation. The concepts inherent in any quality-improvement framework are applicable to all aspects of the nurse manager's role.

> 'The establishment, maintenance, and evaluation of standards of professional nursing practice are central to the role of manager.'

The nature of quality improvement

Health services involve a complex series of related processes from when the person first seeks attention, continuing during the time of admission and treatment, and eventually leading to discharge and community management. The nurse manager has a key role to play in coordinating many of these processes for the benefit of patients.

Quality improvement is a concept that can be applied to all aspects of an organisation. Ideally it should be applied to every process that a health service carries out—from assessment and admission of patients, to carrying out treatment, to discharge and follow-up. It applies to processes as diverse as ensuring that the right procedure is carried out on the right patient at the right time, ensuring that the test results are available in a timely manner, and purchasing and retrieving pharmaceutical supplies.

> 'Quality improvement should be applied to every process that a health service carries out.'

Clinical governance

Clinical governance has been defined as 'the framework through which health organisations are accountable for continuously improving the quality of their services and safeguarding high standards of care by creating an environment in which excellence in clinical care will flourish' (Scally & Donaldson 2001).

Clinical governance involves two fundamental components. First, it involves a commitment from the board of management of the hospital or health service that clinical governance has the same priority as corporate governance—thereby ensuring that effective patient care is as important as ensuring that the books balance. This requires the board to have responsibility for the standards of care delivered in the health service, and for providing the structures and environment in which the delivery of high-quality care can be facilitated. Secondly, clinical governance requires a strong partnership between the board of management and the clinicians—such that all work together to improve patient care.

Such organisational and professional efforts are usually driven by a set of values and the organisation's mission. If an organisation articulates a set of values to guide its work, the behaviour of the organisation should be modelled on the values. For example, an organisation might articulate 'patient-centred' care as a value, and this should be obvious in all aspects of service.

A nurse manager works within this organisational context. Efforts to improve all aspects of service delivery for patient groups need to be aligned with the efforts of the whole organisation, with particular emphasis on professional initiatives that ensure the best healthcare practice is delivered to patients. The nurse manager is therefore an integral part of the clinical governance structure of a health service.

Consumers and customer service

Patients are the reason that health services exist, and are the key drivers of quality.

> Service—the way we treat patients and families in the non-technical components of our interactions with them—has long taken a back seat to medical care. Organizations and clinicians who regard service as unimportant fail to recognize the intimate relationship between clinical outcomes and how people feel about the way we interact with them in all phases of their treatment.
>
> BERWICK (1996)

Consumer interest in health care has increased significantly in recent times. People have become increasingly concerned about standards of care, and increasingly believe that clinicians and organisations should be accountable for services provided (Vincent, Young & Phillips 1994). With the advent of more easily available health information, especially through the Internet, consumers are asserting a more active role in their own health care. This requires health professionals to form more effective partnerships with consumers.

Beginning the process

Initially, the nurse manager and his or her team need to identify the strategic directions and key priorities of the organisation. Some of these will be found in the strategic plan, whereas others will be documented in the last accreditation survey results. The team should also review any data or information that already exists—such as patient or staff incidents, patient feedback, professional development needs, equipment needs, and the results of audits. From these, the team can identify the priorities for its service area, and can formulate relevant goals for the next year. These goals form the basis of the annual 'quality plan' (sometimes called the 'business plan'). This process ensures that the aims of employees, units, and departments are all aligned with the goals of the organisation.

Working with the team, the nurse manager allocates responsibility and timelines to appropriate persons for each initiative. These tasks can also be incorporated into performance-management and staff-development processes. For example, a medical ward might have the goal of implementing primary nursing to support care coordination. Ward nurses might each be required to prepare a nursing-care plan that focuses on the education and empowerment of patients with chronic disabilities, as well as arranging community support services for those people. Nurses might also be expected to improve their own knowledge of the social models for the management of chronic diseases. In this way, the quality-improvement goals of the organisation ultimately reach and improve the health of the customer—the patient.

The next step is to address the system or process that is to be improved. One method that has proved to be very successful for such quality-improvement projects is the 'Plan, Do, Study, Act' (PDSA) cycle (Berwick 1996). These steps are explored in greater detail below.

The PDSA cycle

One method that has proved to be very successful for quality-improvement projects is the PDSA cycle (Berwick 1996). The letters stand for:

- plan;
- do;
- study; and
- act.

These steps are explored in greater detail in the text and form a framework for discussing quality improvement in this chapter.

Plan

Defining the problem

When a team has identified a quality-improvement initiative, the first step is to define the problem clearly.

To take an example, perhaps it has been determined that the incidence of pressure injuries in the ward could be decreased. The actual incidence and the desired incidence must first be established. A clinical audit will indicate the actual incidence, and a perusal of the literature will indicate the desired incidence. For the purposes of this example, it is assumed that the audit shows that, according to a pressure area assessment chart, 20% of patients in the ward have some form of pressure damage, and that a literature review indicates that a desirable level is 5%.

Setting goals

Having defined the problem, the next step is to define a clear goal for the project. The goal needs to be specific, measurable, appropriate, result-oriented, and time-scheduled ('SMART'). In the above example, the goal might be expressed in the following terms: 'To reduce, within two months, the incidence of pressure injuries occurring on the ward from 20% to 5%'.

Other examples of SMART goals in other clinical problems might be as follows.

- 'To reduce by 80%, within one month, the incidence of patients experiencing two or more consecutive days with an international normalised ratio (INR) of greater than 5.'
- 'To eliminate, within three months, the occurrence of wrong tests or wrong procedures being performed on patients.'

Understanding why the problem is occurring

Having defined the problem, and having decided on the 'SMART' goal, the next step is to try to understand *why* the problem is occurring. There are several tools and techniques that can be used for this. These include:

▶ flow charts;
▶ brainstorming;
▶ fishbone diagrams; and
▶ Pareto charts.

Flow charts

Flow charts are a visual representation of the steps or sequences of a process (Brassard & Ritter 1994). Creating a flow chart (often called 'process-mapping') helps people to come to a common understanding of the details of the process.

> 'It is likely that the patient is the only person who ever sees the whole process from beginning to end.'

Many teams are surprised by the complexity of a process once it is actually mapped out—because each individual usually knows about, or works in, only one part of the process. It is likely that the patient is the only person who ever sees the whole process from beginning to end. The very act of creating the flow chart can often help to clarify some of the weaknesses of a system and how it can be improved or simplified.

The first flow chart that should be drawn is called a 'high-level chart'. This might require only 4–5 steps to describe the overall process. For example, the high-level flow chart of the patient-identification process shown in Figure 12.1 (page 135) has six major steps in ensuring that the right patient gets the right investigation or treatment. A more detailed or low-level flow chart shows the many steps that are actually involved in transporting the right patient to the appropriate place for the procedure.

Brainstorming

When it is important to generate as many ideas as possible, brainstorming is a good technique to use (Brassard & Ritter 1994). The group involved in the issue should meet and take the following steps:

▶ appoint a scribe;
▶ write the problem or question on a flip chart or board;
▶ ensure that everyone understands the topic and the rules;

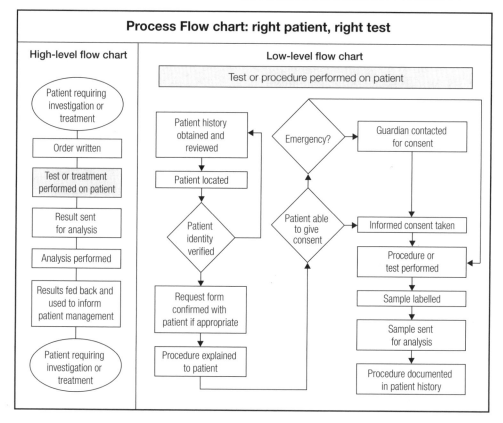

Figure 12.1 Process flow chart: right patient, right test
Authors' creation

▸ ensure that every team member has an opportunity to suggest an idea on
'post-it' notes, a board, or a flip chart;
▸ stop before fatigue sets in;
▸ review the list and eliminate duplicates; and
▸ group ideas by common themes.

Fishbone diagrams (cause-and-effect diagrams)

When utilising a team approach to problem-solving, there are often many
opinions about the problem's root cause. One way to capture these different ideas
and to stimulate the team's brainstorming is a cause-and-effect diagram
(commonly called a 'fishbone diagram') (Brassard & Ritter 1994).

A fishbone diagram helps to display the many potential causes for a specific
problem or effect. It is particularly useful in a group setting and for situations in
which little quantitative data are available for analysis.

To construct a fishbone diagram, the problem should be stated in the form of a question, such as: 'Why might patients receive too much warfarin?'. Framing the problem as a 'why' question assists analysis and brainstorming—because each 'root cause' idea that is subsequently proposed should answer the initial 'why' question.

The team should agree on the statement of the problem, and then place this question in a box at the 'head' of the fishbone. Figure 12.2 (below) shows an example of a fishbone diagram used in a hospital setting to analyse the reasons for patients receiving an incorrect dose of warfarin.

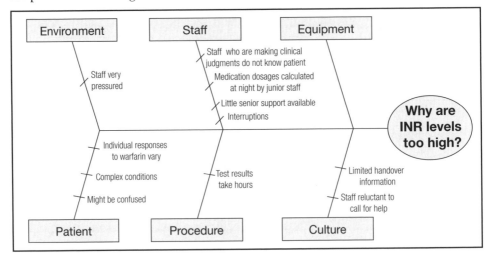

Figure 12.2 Fishbone analysis for incorrect warfarin dosage
Authors' creation

Pareto charts

A Pareto chart can be used to help prioritise actions (Brassard & Ritter 1994). The Pareto principle is that 'a minority of input produces the majority of results'. This is often expressed in shorthand form as the '80–20 rule'—that 80% of all problems are caused by 20% of all possible causes of those problems. Therefore, if the most common causes of a given problem can be identified and addressed, it is likely that most of the problem can be eliminated.

'If the most common causes of a given problem can be addressed, it is likely that most of the problem can be eliminated.'

For example, if the nursing staff decided to survey the junior medical staff to determine their perceptions of the reasons for inappropriate warfarin dosages, the junior medical staff's responses could be presented as shown in Table 12.1 below.

Table 12.1 Initial survey data

Problems leading to inaccurate warfarin dosages (as identified by house medical officers)	% of responses	Why?
1. INR/warfarin after-hours cover	29	prescribed by evening shift
2. Forgetting to write 'stat' order	19	prescribed by evening shift
3. Recalling which patient is on warfarin	16	prescribed by evening shift
4. INR result not available by 1700 hrs	14	current practice in pathology
5. Forgetting to order INR	10	prescribed by evening shift
6. Forgetting to review INR result	7	prescribed by evening shift
7. Lack of knowledge	4	insufficient education

Authors' creation

Having determined the factors most likely to contribute to the problem, the next step is to ask 'Why?' as many times as is necessary to get to the bottom of the issue. In the case of incorrect warfarin dosages, the team might identify that many of the issues arose because the patient had complex medical problems. However, the doctors who note the INR results and prescribe the next warfarin dose are likely to be junior medical staff on the evening shift who do not know the patients, have minimal handover, and have little experience.

If the survey findings are then graphed from highest frequency to lowest frequency, a Pareto chart can be formed, as shown in Figure 12.3 (page 138). Using this information, the team is then able to conclude that the doctors on the day shift should be responsible for prescribing the evening warfarin dosages if the outcome for patients is to be improved.

Do

As noted above (page 133), one method that has proved to be very successful for quality-improvement projects is the 'Plan, Do, Study, Act' (PDSA) cycle (Berwick 1996). Having completed the first step ('Plan'), the next step is to proceed to the second step ('Do) by carrying out the plan.

In the warfarin case study, the team might decide to move the time of warfarin administration to 4 pm—before the end of the day shift. This would ensure that the doctors prescribing the dosages were the same doctors who routinely cared for the patients. To do this, the team would have to ensure that the pathology test results were available by lunchtime each day.

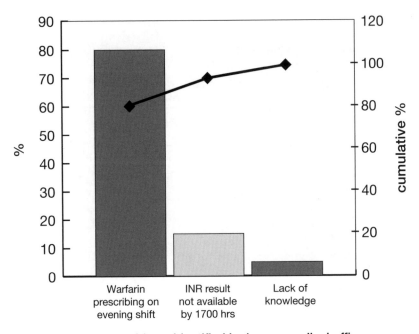

Figure 12.3 Pareto chart: problems identified by house medical officers
Authors' creation

Implementing this change would require education and good communication among all staff members involved to ensure that the prescription of warfarin dosages took place at 4 pm, and that any obstacles to this change were overcome as soon as possible.

As in all improvement initiatives, it is important that the interventions agreed are clearly detailed and that responsibilities are assigned.

Study

The next step in 'Plan, Do, Study, Act' (PDSA) cycle (Berwick 1996) is to *study* the results. Simple, easy-to-obtain measures can be used to monitor the results of interventions. These can be samples or indicators of the problem. Trying to collect perfect, comprehensive data is a common reason for quality-improvement teams floundering at this stage. Figure 12.4 (page 139) shows initial outcome data for the warfarin prescribing problem under discussion.

Change in prescribing time leads to improved warfarin levels

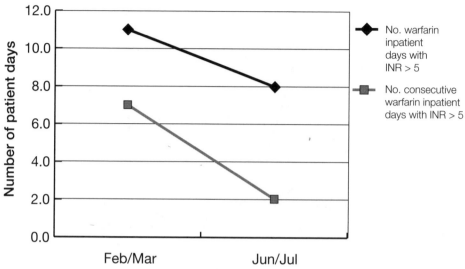

Figure 12.4 Initial outcome data
Authors' creation

The team should then ask what changed and whether this was an improvement. In the warfarin project, the team would conclude that it had significantly improved the problem. However, feedback might indicate that staff members require reminders to continue the new arrangements—for example, the junior doctors might require reminders to check the INR results and prescribe at the appropriate time.

Act

The final step in the 'Plan, Do, Study, Act' (PDSA) cycle (Berwick 1996) is to *act* on the study of results. To continue to improve the process, the team in this case study might introduce a 'memory jogger' to alert staff members who manage patients on warfarin. An alert sticker reading 'warfarin 4 pm' could be placed on the patient's history.

The team should continue to reinforce the safe warfarin strategy by providing feedback of warfarin survey results to medical, nursing, and pharmacy staff, and by distributing a 'warfarin 4 pm' alert sticker to wards and the doctors' lounge.

As a result of this project, the usage of warfarin might be expected to improve dramatically, with better outcomes for patients (see Figure 12.5, page 140).

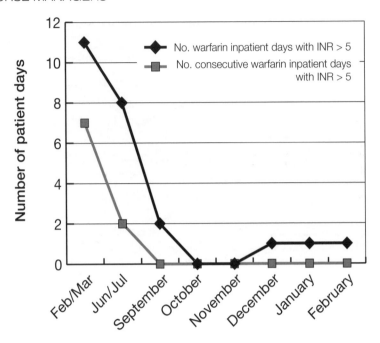

Figure 12.5 Final outcome data
Authors' creation

Storyboards

A 'storyboard' (also known as a 'brag board') is a simple summary of a quality-improvement project. Placed on a board or poster, it commends quality-improvement initiatives, and thereby encourages other similar projects.

Storyboards should (Leape et al. 2000):

▶ be designed for ease of comprehension and readability;
▶ include only critical information;
▶ be kept simple;
▶ make the purpose of the investigation readily apparent;
▶ describe interventions concisely;
▶ display data over time using control charts; and
▶ outline conclusions based upon data.

Sustaining improvements

Creating and sustaining improvements in a service is one of the most challenging and rewarding tasks for managers.

Research of 'human factors' enables managers to gain an understanding of how people perform in the workplace—both individually and in teams. The key finding of this type of research is that people perform tasks well when individuals have the necessary skills and desires, and when the system in which they work supports their best performance. In the case of the safe warfarin project, staff members wanted their patients to have the correct INR levels. The team therefore changed the system to ensure that the INR results were available earlier, and that the doctors prescribing the warfarin dosages knew the patients well.

> 'People perform tasks well when . . . the system in which they work supports their best performance.'

The Box below summarises some tips for success in quality-improvement projects.

Tips for success

The following points have been identified as fundamental in gaining quality improvement.

- Nurses should concentrate on meeting the needs of patients rather than the needs of the organisation.
- The more specific the aim, the more likely an improvement will result.
- Real improvement comes from changing systems, not changing from within systems.
- Not all change is improvement, but all improvement is change.
- Measurement helps: (i) to determine whether innovations should be kept, changed, or rejected; (ii) to understand causes; and (iii) to clarify aims.
- To make improvement there must be clarity as to what is to be accomplished, how it will be recognised when a change has led to an improvement, and what change can be made that will lead to an improvement.

Adapted from Berwick (1996)

Effective leaders challenge the status quo by insisting that the current system must be changed, and by offering clear ideas about superior alternatives.

Concepts that should be incorporated into the improvements are:
- reducing reliance on memory;
- simplifying and standardising;
- using constraints and forcing functions;
- using protocols and checklists wisely;

▶ improving information access;
▶ decreasing reliance on vigilance;
▶ reducing hand-offs and increasing feedback;
▶ decreasing multiple entry and look-alikes; and
▶ automating carefully.

Above all, collaboration with other clinical leaders and other service providers—such as quality-and-safety units, information technology, health-information services, and medical and allied health services—increases the chances of success.

Conclusion

Continuously striving to improve the quality and safety of the health service provided by a team is a key function of a nurse manager. To do this, it is necessary to understand the role of the nurse manager in the clinical governance of the organisation, be familiar with the organisation's strategic directions, and lead the team using simple tools to measure, analyse, and improve the care given to patients.

Chapter 13

Writing Policies and Procedures

Neil Croll

Introduction

There are basically two sorts of policies—*public* policy (at the level of government) and *organisational* policy (at the level of a particular healthcare service). Despite its importance, *public* policy has never been defined in a way that is universally accepted. Perhaps this is because the term is used to describe a number of apparently different activities. These include (Hogwood & Gunn 1984):

- a label for a field of government activity;
- an expression of general purpose or desired state of affairs;
- specific proposals;
- decisions of government;
- formal authorisation;
- programs;
- output;
- outcome;
- theory or model; and
- process.

Each of these aspects of *public* policy can be translated to an area of *organisational* policy by a health service.

The first, *a label for a field of government activity*, can be translated to various types of organisational activity—such as management, clinical services, hotel services, engineering, and information technology.

The second, *an expression of general purpose or desired state of affairs*, could include any of the pamphlets or other information that a hospital produces to tell people about its services. Usually, such information tells people what they can expect from the health service, without specifying how many people it will service or how much better they will become as a result.

Specific proposals could include such plans as the establishment of a 'Centre for Older People's Health', including health-promotion and health-monitoring programs. Such proposals would be much more detailed than expressions of general purpose.

Decisions of government clearly translates as 'decisions of the health service'. This does not mean only the decisions written down and called 'policy decisions', but also refers to a wide range of decisions that might include memoranda, explanations, and minutes of committees.

Formal authorisation means the decisions that bear the official authority of the organisation. A health service might put up notices prohibiting smoking anywhere in the buildings, on the grounds, or in any vehicles. Such notices might have a line at the bottom that reads something like: 'Authorised by the Board of Management, M. Smithers, Chief Executive Officer'. A written policy to say that smoking is banned might not exist, but such formal authorisation is enough to convey that this is effectively the policy of the organisation.

Programs are areas of activity. A health service might have general medical and surgical programs, as well as programs for obstetrics, orthopaedics, mental health, and community nursing. The existence of these programs represents a policy of the organisation.

Output is a quantitative measure. For example, an output target might be set for a day-surgery program and be expressed as a certain number of operations per month, based on similar data from other units that do the same sort of work.

Outcome is a qualitative measure. Whereas *output* asks how *many* of something will be achieved, *outcome* asks how *well* it will be done. For example, a target output might be set for 20 knee reconstructions per week, but if the infection rate is 28%, or if people experience less mobility after their operations than before, the outcome is not at all good.

Theory or model refers to an underlying idea or set of ideas that determine how decisions are made. Many health services are operated by religious organisations and openly state that they follow the ideals of that particular religion. In other cases the model might not be openly stated, but examination of the decisions that have been made might provide evidence of a pattern that adds up to such a model of belief.

Process means *how* something is to be done, rather than *what* it is to achieve. Processes go well beyond procedures. They include organisational structures, networks of committees, auditing details, and pathways of information.

In summary, *policies* are decisions about what is to be achieved, how it is to be achieved, how resources will be used, how the organisation will handle things that go wrong, and how it will ensure that things do not go wrong too often. Policies are thus decisions that affect large numbers of cases rather than single events, and they represent how the organisation wishes to be perceived by people examining its operations from the outside. In contrast, a *procedure* is the specific way of doing something that ensures that policies are met.

> 'Policies are decisions about what is to be achieved . . . a procedure is the specific way of doing something that ensures that policies are met.'

Importance of policies

Most healthcare professionals are familiar with manuals of *policy* and *procedure* in health services, but it is wrong to assume that everything that is included in such manuals represents consistent policy or procedure. An examination of the procedures of an organisation might reveal that it has many unstated policies that have never been officially documented and authorised. Indeed, if organisational procedures are analysed, it might become apparent that a health service has policies that are quite different from those it claims to have.

Consistent and known policies are critically important to organisations for several reasons. Such policies:

▶ enable decisions to be predictable and fair to all, rather than being capricious and biased;

▶ save time (and therefore money) that would have to be spent making case-by-case decisions;

▶ enable the operations of the organisation to be open and transparent;

▶ can be revised to keep up with developments in best practice, technical advances, laws and regulations, and the requirements of external organisations (such as professional boards);

❱ meet many of the demands of accreditation processes; and
❱ can give legal protection to staff members against allegations
   of malpractice.

However, these benefits will follow only if the policies are well developed and well written, and if they are kept current and not allowed to become obsolete.

Policy framework

In deciding which policy areas are needed, it is advisable to work from the broadest policy first. A broad structure is needed before the fine details can be filled in. The first policy might therefore be called 'Framework for service' or 'Management and structure'—thus representing a framework for the entire service. This might include things such as the mission and vision statements, the organisational framework (the divisions and departments), the management structure, and the structure of committees and their terms of reference (including what they are excluded from doing). One of the items in this early section might well be a statement on policy development itself. This could outline the process by which policies are written, scrutinised, authorised, and applied in the workplace.

'A broad structure is needed before the fine details can be filled in.'

The scope of such a policy framework requires careful attention. One area worthy of inclusion might be the *environment* in which the service is delivered. How should the organisation ensure that the working environment is safe for staff members and patients? This section could include occupational health and safety, infection control, and emergency management. Another area worthy of inclusion might be *practice*—that is, the way in which service is actually delivered to patients. This could include general policy on how various treatments are to be delivered.

The policy framework needs to take account of the requirements of other authorities and organisations. These might include:

❱ professional registration bodies;
❱ national healthcare standards;
❱ professional organisations;
❱ statute and common law;
❱ accreditation organisations;
❱ funding organisations;
❱ government policy;

▶ local building regulations;
▶ insurance companies; and
▶ unions.

For example, an accreditation body might specify that the service should have a policy relating to the access of its facilities by other organisations, or a funding organisation might prescribe the data that should be collected on the programs that it funds. Some of the demands of these various organisations could well be contradictory.

Policy development

Once an organisation has its basic policy framework in place, it is in a position to develop and implement specific policies. For this, a structure is needed through which to work.

Most organisations have a committee for policy and procedure. This committee is constituted to generate policies and procedures, and to pass them to the board of management and/or the chief executive officer for authorisation and implementation. Care is needed in constituting the membership of such a committee. Departmental managers who have the authority to make decisions on

'If the committee is too large it will take too long to make decisions, the process will be slow, and the decisions might be out of date before they can be applied.'

behalf of the main sections of the organisation are needed on such a committee, but if the committee is too large it will take too long to make decisions, the process will be slow, and the decisions might be out of date before they can be applied.

In larger organisations, individual departments might well need their own policy-development committees or working groups to develop policies that are then presented to the organisational policy-and-procedure committee for ratification. Given that policies represent the current best practice in each area, local experts need to be able to research latest developments and give specialist technical advice.

At the lower levels of an organisation, policy development can become problematic. For some years the concept of workplace democracy has been accepted as desirable, even mandatory. However, a process whereby all employees have a voice in the policy decisions (or any other decisions) is time-consuming and costly, and does not guarantee the best results. There is a strong

> 'It is desirable that employees "own" decisions because this is more likely to result in compliance.'

risk of self-interest taking precedence over organisational strategy, and 'on-the-ground' employees are often disconnected from the larger strategic landscape in which the organisation operates. However, it is desirable that employees 'own' decisions because this is more likely to result in compliance. Staff meetings are good opportunities for consultation about proposed policies.

Policy implementation

After policies have been developed and authorised, the question arises as to how they are to be implemented.

Most statements of duty (as detailed in position or job descriptions) require staff members to practise in accordance with organisational policies, but a court of law might not consider it reasonable for an organisation to implement policies without a mechanism for informing its staff of the changes. The terms of reference for staff meetings should therefore require that all memoranda and notices are listed in the minutes, attached to the published minutes, or posted on noticeboards. This gives all affected staff members an opportunity to be aware of changes.

Some organisations go so far as to require all staff members to read new policies, and to sign a statement that they have read, understood, and are now bound by the provisions.

Content of policies

Policy documents should be presented with clearly defined headings as follows:
▶ introduction (or preamble);
▶ the policy itself;
▶ statement of responsibility;
▶ authorisation;
▶ dates of application and review; and
▶ references.

Each of these is discussed below.

The *introduction* is a statement of what the policy is all about. It should be expressed in the simplest possible terms without being too specific. The aim of this section is to tell the reader whether this is the policy that he or she is looking for, and whether to read on for more detail.

The *policy* itself is the main statement that sets out what is required, and how the organisation should do it. A decision needs to be made as to how specific this statement should be. Outcome measures might be included to enable future determinations to be made about whether the policy worked, how well it worked, and how staff performed in implementing the policy.

The *statement of responsibility* outlines those to whom the policy applies. For example, it should state whether the policy applies to all staff members or only to nurses; or whether the policy applies to all sections within a department, or only to one section. A general principle to follow is that policies should apply to as many people in the organisation as possible. If different departments have separate policies to define standards, management should consider whether one policy could apply to these various staff groups.

The *authorisation* of a policy is very important. Policies cannot be written and adopted by just anybody; they need to be authorised by the appropriate person or committee. Usually, policies are authorised by the chief executive officer of the organisation on behalf of the board of management. It is not acceptable for the chairperson of the board to authorise policies because the chairperson might not be legally accountable for such decisions. Such authority is therefore usually delegated to the chief executive officer. Depending on the organisational structure (which is, in itself, another policy), policy authorisation might be delegated to a committee or a particular person in a division or department—in which case it has authority only in that section of the organisation.

Content of policy documents

Policy documents should be presented with clearly defined headings as follows:
- introduction (or preamble);
- the policy itself;
- statement of responsibility;
- authorisation;
- dates of application and review; and
- references.

The *dates of application and review* validate the policy. Over time an organisation is likely to generate several 'generations' of policies, and there must be some way of knowing which document is currently in force. The date of authorisation must therefore be stated. Policy frameworks are constantly evolving to adapt to all sorts of conditions. Policies are thus 'living documents' that are constantly under review to ensure that they reflect the current realities in health services.

References in policy documents point to sources of material contained in the policy, and to other sources of material that support the policy. For example, a medication policy might contain cross-references to the following supporting information:

- regulations of the nurse-registration authority;
- statutory Acts governing medication administration;
- statements of professional organisations on medication policy;
- accreditation standards; and
- other policies and procedures within the organisation's own framework.

The references add to the authority of the policy.

Policy documents

Policy documents should be carefully prepared in the knowledge that they will be read by various people. These include staff members of the organisation, people inspecting the service for purposes of accreditation, various other people from outside the organisation who make judgments about the quality of the service, and, possibly, lawyers looking for ways to prosecute or defend charges against the organisation. The documents should therefore be carefully crafted before they are authorised and distributed.

> 'Policy documents should be carefully crafted before they are authorised and distributed.'

Drafting policy documents is much easier if computer files have been set up with a standardised format adopted by the organisation. Some guidelines for such a document format are:

- define the standardised style by setting up a blank template file (including fonts, point sizes, indents, margins, gutters, and alignment rules);
- define the language rules (for example, which dictionary is to be followed, and how formal the expression will be);
- insert page numbers automatically;
- insert the author's name, the file name, and the pathway automatically (either as a footer in the whole file, or on the last page); and
- set out all the sections needed (for example, introduction, policy, responsibility, authorisation, and references).

Health services produce many documents designed for public consumption, and often find great benefit from using professional editors from within their organisations or from external companies. Adoption of a 'house style' (even if the style varies depending on the application of the document) provides uniformity to public documents and enables readers to identify with the style of the organisation.

As with any documentation, the readers must be carefully considered. The language used must be clearly understandable to those to whom the policy applies, and this can mean that some variation is required for different sections. For example, different terminology might be required in various sections that are directed specifically to doctors, or to nurses, or to other categories of staff. Consideration should also be given to the terms that are habitually used by various organisations.

> 'With any documentation, the readers must be carefully considered.'

In addition to a 'house style', a set of 'house abbreviations' is useful to ensure that there is no confusion regarding the meanings attached to various terms and acronyms.

Safeguards in policy development

Some thought should be given to having the policy drafts scrutinised by experts. This can avoid the inclusion or exclusion of matters that might cause trouble later. Such experts might include the quality-control manager, the clinical-risk manager, the human-resources manager, and a legal advisor. Depending on the particular policy being drafted, the engineering department, the public-relations officer, and other departments that are incidentally affected by the policy should be consulted.

It is useful to keep a record of the processes followed. This provides evidence to support the authority of the policy (if this is needed).

Management of policies

Many organisations simply collect policies into loose-leaf folders. But this is usually inadequate for storage and access. Most heath services have too many policies containing too much information to make this a practical choice. Rather than present people with huge folders of inaccessible information, policy collections should be divided into sections that allow people to select the section of the collection that applies to them.

Computers provide the best means of storing information in a way that allows users to navigate straight to the information required without wasting time. Almost all policy documents are produced on word-processors, and these documents can be loaded onto the service's Intranet site as word-processing files. However, it is important to ensure that people cannot alter the files. This can be overcome by using portable document format (pdf) for storage. Such pdf files have the added advantage of being smaller than most word-processing files.

Navigational tools can be added to the Intranet policy collection. This should begin with a contents file that lists each policy on the file server, along with the dates authorised and the review dates. Each policy entry in the list of contents can be hyperlinked to the file that contains the policy itself.

Conclusion

Policies, and the procedures that specify exactly how policy goals are to be achieved, should be part of a considered decision-making framework. Such a framework facilitates high standards of service provision, provides safeguards against legal actions, ensures economy, fairness, consistency in decision-making, and enhances interfaces between health services and other organisations.

Policies and procedures should be carefully crafted after adequate research has been carried out to ensure that they meet the requirements of the organisation and satisfy the various demands that are placed on the service by outside organisations.

A carefully researched and crafted framework for policy and procedural development is a most worthwhile investment in quality processes and outcomes.

Chapter 14

Working with Job Descriptions

Greg Price

Introduction

Job descriptions (or *position descriptions*) play a vital role in the success of organisational performance. They provide a clear written template of roles and expected performance for both an organisation and for individual employees.

At the recruitment phase, a job or position description gives a prospective employee an opportunity for self-assessment of suitability. In a sense this represents the commencement of the culling phase of selection. Throughout the period of employment the description serves as a basis for performance evaluation, as well as for position review and position redesign. In the post-employment phase, the description can be further reviewed and refined to assist the organisation to achieve its goals.

Recruitment

The major components of a job or position description are generally written in a summarised format for job advertisements. Interested applicants usually then apply for an employment package that includes a role description and/or person specification. The position description details the requirements of the role whereas the person specification relates some of the personal attributes that are sought.

Ongoing employment

All employees, new and existing, should have a current job or position description. This means that ongoing formal review of all position descriptions must be undertaken as a routine function of management. Organisations are subject to constant changes—not only in the turnover of personnel, but also in relation to technology and legislation—and it is important to ensure that long-term employees are routinely kept in touch with the needs of the organisation by receiving updated job or position descriptions.

> 'All employees, new and existing, should have a current job or position description.'

Main components
Standard template

An agreed layout and content of the job or position description should be established, and a standard template should be agreed for use throughout the organisation. It is important to use simple language in the description. Standardisation and simplicity minimise confusion and reduce possible misinterpretations.

> 'Standardisation and simplicity minimise confusion and reduce possible misinterpretations.'

Assessing currency

There are several ways to assess the currency of the design and content. The wider health marketplace can be used by simply applying for employment packages to see how it is done elsewhere. Approaches can also be made to an employers' association, or a professional set of personnel documentation guidelines can be purchased.

Example of a template

A general template for a job or position description for a registered nurse might read as shown in the Box below.

General template for a job or position description

Organisational heading

The organisation states its name and location. This can include the organisation's logo. If included, the logo serves to build a symbolic relationship between the organisation and the employee.

Job or position description

(i) Title

This describes the role that the person will be required to fill. The title can be worded carefully to reflect the nature of the position; for example, 'quality coordinator'.

(ii) Award classification

This relates the position to the relevant award classification; for example, registered nurse.

Terms and conditions of employment

This might be stated simply as being 'per the relevant award' (with the name of the award being stated).

Department (or section)

This confirms the physical area in which the employee is required to work; for example, oncology ward.

Responsible to

This reflects the line of authority as detailed in the organisation chart; for example, director of nursing.

Hours per week

This states the number of hours that the person is contracted to work. Alternatively, this can be set out in the employment contract.

Performance appraisal

If a statement of the appraisal arrangements is included, initial appraisal should be conducted three months after commencement date, and then annually using the position description and agreed performance objectives.

Purpose of the position

This might include a statement that binds the position to the philosophy and objectives of the organisation; for example: 'This registered nurse position is a fundamental part of a management system that is designed to ensure the professional and responsible management of nursing-service delivery in a manner that is consistent with the philosophy, objectives, and policies of the organisation.'

(Continued)

(*Continued*)

Such a statement is useful in providing a framework for understanding why the position has been constructed.

Body of the description

The formulation of the position description should be based upon the philosophy and objectives of the organisation.

There is no right or wrong way of writing the body of a job or position description. One approach is to divide the description into two major columns. The left-hand column lists major performance standards whereas the right-hand column provides specific key performance indicators of each performance standard.

Extra information

Management might wish to provide supplementary information. This can be included as an attachment to the position description, or it can be included in the orientation manual.

The extra information elaborates on the role as part of the broader management framework. In its simplest form this might simply state:

- that the job or position description forms a part of the recruitment, selection, and appraisal process;
- that it is routinely updated; and
- that staff members are required to sign two copies of the description (with each party retaining a copy for further reference).

Person specification

A person specification is usually included to supplement the position description. This is particularly useful at the pre-employment stage. It assists prospective employees to gain knowledge about the type of person that the organisation seeks in terms of qualifications, skills, experience, and abilities. A person specification can also include personality attributes—such as empathy, effective communication skills, helpfulness, and so on.

Relationship between organisation and individual

The job or position description plays an important role in communicating the expectations of the organisation and should assist employees by providing easy-to-understand performance guidelines. This serves to bond employees and the organisation into a partnership of mutual understanding.

However, there is always a formal interface between the characteristics of an individual employee and the formal requirements of the organisation. Because people are individuals—each with a personal set of skills, experiences, and personalities—a balance between flexibility and autocracy must be maintained.

The degree of flexibility depends upon the nature of the position.

Positions that involve a lot of predictable work in a stable environment infer a more autocratic arrangement in which guidelines clearly set out the exact performances that are expected. Examples of these types of positions include task-related or process-related duties such as those that occur in domestic services, care delivery, and clerical jobs.

Positions that are less predictable have greater flexibility, and in these roles a *formal* job or position description might gradually evolve into an *informal* description. However, there are inherent difficulties in such informal arrangements.

If it becomes apparent that some staff members perform their duties as if they do not know what they are doing, the nurse manager should pause and think—perhaps it is because they do *not* know what they are supposed to be doing! This can occur if some activities have not been allocated. In these circumstances, staff members gradually 'fill the gap'. It can also occur if staff members have forgotten exactly what they are supposed to do.

> 'If staff members perform their duties as if they do not know what they are doing, perhaps it is because they do *not* know what they are supposed to be doing!'

There will always be some element of discrepancy between what is done and what is expected. However, routine review processes help to uncover these. If such routine reviews do not occur, the organisation runs the risk of becoming dysfunctional. Regular reviews should therefore be conducted.

Duty guides

Management can also provide guidance in everyday activities by issuing duty guides. These give general instructions regarding the tasks and routine activities to be undertaken. The Box on page 158 provides an example of an extract from a duty guide for a registered nurse in an aged-care facility.

In the example given in the Box, the role of the registered nurse is a middle-management position. The duties involve coordinating and managing the activities of a group of nurses. A position description at this level combines elements of autocracy with elements of flexibility.

Example of a duty guide for a registered nurse

7.00 am
- commence duty
- receive report from night duty
- check roster allocations and staff levels
- check diary regarding appointments
- check calendar for professional development and/or committee meetings
- check accountable medications
- attend aged-care treatments

7.30 am
- commence medication round
- coordinate nursing activities with allocated staff

9.30 am
- morning tea

9.45 am
- attend to specialised procedures

11.30 am
- attend to lunchtime medications

12.00 noon
- lunch

12.30 pm
- report to oncoming nursing staff

1.00 pm
- continue clinical duties and collect feedback from staff

2.30 pm
- check professional development activities
- attend handover report to evening staff

2.50 pm
- ensure that staff members have completed allocated tasks and that all areas are clean before staff members finish their shifts

3.20 pm
- complete duty

In contrast, at the senior-management level, a duty guide is inappropriate because most actions are fairly flexible. Elements that require prescription can be incorporated directly into the job or position description—for example, 'prepare and submit a monthly report'.

At the levels of lower management, a duty guide becomes increasingly relevant as a supplement to the job or position description. The Box below provides an example of a duty guide for a cleaner.

Example of a duty guide for a cleaner

6.30 am
- commence duty; report to night-duty registered nurse
- clean lounge; empty bins; dry and wet mop
- vacuum main foyer area and common rooms
- review equipment and cleaning stations (ensuring adequate stock)
- clean staff and public toilets; empty bins

9.00 am
- morning tea

9.15 am
- proceed to main nursing wards
- clean bathrooms and toilets
- empty bins
- clean and mop floors

1.00 pm
- lunch

1.30 pm
- check with services manager regarding special duties
- ensure all bathrooms, showers, and toilets are clean
- clean dirty utility rooms (including bench areas and bins)
- clean public toilets
- vacuum foyer area

3.00 pm
- complete duty

Routine reviews

Review of description

A review of job or position descriptions involves an evaluation of the description against the nature of the role. Specific feedback regarding the relevance of the description can occur at formal or informal levels.

Formal review involves quality-improvement processes and structured management tasks. The content of the position is analysed against the current needs of the organisation, and any identified discrepancies are addressed. This usually occurs at scheduled intervals (for example, annually) or when the position becomes vacant. It is especially important to undertake a formal review of low-turnover positions. Other forms of formal review include simple feedback channels (such as a suggestion box, staff surveys, staff interviews, and staff meetings) or a formal staff-appraisal system.

'It is especially important to undertake a formal review of low-turnover positions.'

Informal review involves everyday dialogue between management and staff. It is important that nurse managers be alert to the fact that operational dysfunctions can occur due to poorly written and infrequently reviewed position descriptions.

Performance review and staff appraisal

The job or position description lies within the ambit of performance management. It conveys information to the employee regarding:

❯ the outcomes that the employee must work towards achieving;
❯ the key performance measures of the position; and
❯ the level of performance standard that is required.

The level of performance can be linked to an externally derived standard—such as professionally mandated standards set by accreditation authorities or professional bodies. This ensures adherence with standards of best practice.

The major performance standards and key performance indicators can be directly transcribed into the design of the appraisal tool used by the organisation. This ensures consistency in feedback mechanisms—including self-review, peer-review, and supervisor-review.

Significance of reviews

It is important that the job or position descriptions act as a level playing field for all stakeholders. Management and staff must have a common point of reference. When reviewing position descriptions, management should ensure that the following concepts are addressed:

❯ appropriate appraisal and performance indicators;
❯ opportunities for organisational and individual learning and growth;
❯ the possible utilisation of duty guides to ensure compliance with procedural outcomes;
❯ the role of professional competency frameworks to ensure compliance with professional standards;
❯ the role of legislation and regulatory bodies; and
❯ routine review of *all* job and position descriptions.

The review process might therefore uncover gaps between expected performance and actual performance. In addition, the review process might also uncover anomalies in the job or position description itself.

The job or position description thus provides a basis for both individual development and organisational development.

Conclusion

Management cannot reasonably expect staff to meet required performance levels unless these are clearly set out for the employee's reference. This is especially relevant at the commencement of employment.

In addition, a job or position description provides organisational continuity of purpose in managing the diversity of people within the organisation.

Such descriptions should therefore be based on a recent assessment of the effectiveness and efficiency of work practices (rather than being retrieved from the bottom drawer of a filing cabinet), and should be circulated among existing staff to ensure that existing staff members and more recently recruited staff do not have different perceptions of their roles.

Chapter 15

Selecting, Recruiting, and Retaining Staff

Neville Phillips

Introduction

The selecting, recruiting, and retaining of quality nurses is now a critical activity for health services. Nursing shortages are not new and, until recently, have been perceived as inevitable events in the cycle of supply and demand. However, the current shortage of nurses is a worldwide problem, rather than a local phenomenon. The present worldwide shortage is '. . . quite different as no recovery is projected' (Fitzgerald 2002, p. 109).

Nurses rightfully see themselves as a valuable and scarce resource and, when recruiting and retaining new nurses, the nurse manager requires processes that are robust and creative if they are to ensure a good match between individual nurses and the positions to be filled.

Recruitment and retention are inextricably linked. Employers who have a reputation for sound employment practices and who actively seek to retain quality staff are attractive choices for nurses who wish to be recruited. Furthermore, retention is improved by effective recruitment processes that maximise job satisfaction by matching nurses' skills and preferences to vacant positions.

Selection and recruitment

When confronted with filling a nursing vacancy, many nurse managers view the recruitment process as merely another bureaucratic demand that they must squeeze into an already full schedule. In fact, recruitment is one of the most important tasks that the nurse manager undertakes on behalf of a health service and, ultimately, on behalf of the people whom the service exists to serve.

A positive match of the right person with the right job improves the quality of services. At best, a poor match can mean undertaking the whole process again; at worst, depending on industrial and human-resource environments, a poor match can mean a protracted and damaging process of having to remove or reassign a nurse.

An effective recruitment process involves 13 steps:
- completing a position review;
- reviewing the job description and person specification;
- having the position checked;
- advertising the position;
- establishing the selection panel;
- shortlisting the candidates;
- undertaking a selection process;
- conducting the interview;
- checking references;
- making the decision;
- writing the selection report;
- informing the candidates; and
- inducting the successful candidate.

Each of these is discussed below.

1. Completing a position review

Few positions within modern health services remain static. Therefore, the first step in the recruitment process is to have a clear view of the demands of the vacant position and the attributes required of the person who is to fill it. In reviewing a position, the nurse manager should seek out as many sources of information as possible—including speaking with nurses in similar roles in other health services and seeking feedback from other staff members who relate to the position.

If there is advance notice of an imminent vacancy, the present post-holder should be asked to keep a log of daily activity. Alternatively, the nurse manager might spend some time observing the work of the present post-holder. Previous employees are often one of the most reliable sources of information. Any exit interviews should be reviewed and a new exit interview conducted with the post-holder. Available performance appraisals should also be referred to.

In addition to reviewing the role as it exists, the nurse manager should also review expectations of how the role will evolve over time. Questions to be asked include:

▶ Does the position fit with the organisation's strategic plan?

▶ What are the medium-term and long-term expectations for the position?

▶ How should the consumer of the service influence the position design?

Finally, any associated documentation relevant to the position should be reviewed—such as duty statements, or policies and procedures.

An effective recruitment process

An effective recruitment process involves 13 steps:
- completing a position review;
- reviewing the job description and person specification;
- having the position checked;
- advertising the position;
- establishing the selection panel;
- shortlisting the candidates;
- undertaking a selection process;
- conducting the interview;
- checking references;
- making the decision;
- writing the selection report;
- informing the candidates; and
- inducting the successful candidate.

A discussion of these steps forms the framework of this section of the chapter.

---

2. Reviewing the job description and person specification

Job descriptions should be written in a style that clearly describes the activities and relationships that are required to achieve the outcomes identified in the review of the position described in Step 1. Activities should be listed in order of priority, and descriptions of those activities should state how the achievement of the role's purpose will be measured.

'Job descriptions should be written in a style that clearly describes the activities and relationships that are required to achieve the outcomes identified.'

These descriptions should be realistic and should not be constructed in such a way that few nurses (if any) can fulfil them.

Person specifications should describe the characteristics that a nurse needs to possess to achieve the activities required in the position. These characteristics are often written in terms of: (i) *absolute* or *essential* characteristics (that are crucial to the achievement of the role); and (ii) *desirable* or *preferred* characteristics (that are not critical, but would add to the success of the role).

Characteristics are typically categorised as 'skills', 'knowledge', and 'personal attributes'. In drawing up a list of desirable characteristics, the nurse manager should avoid being too exhaustive, and should keep to key characteristics. Of all the possible characteristics, attention should especially be paid to:

- enthusiasm;
- creativity;
- leadership;
- ability to perform under pressure;
- flexibility;
- decision-making;
- the ability to work in a team;
- communication skills;
- business management skills; and
- client advocacy.

Nurse managers should be aware of certain skills or knowledge that a nurse could easily obtain *after* appointment. It is important not to exclude a quality candidate merely because one particular experience or skill is absent.

> 'Nurse managers should be aware of certain skills or knowledge that a nurse could easily obtain *after* appointment.'

A key requirement when preparing person specifications is to decide how a nurse might be expected to demonstrate any particular characteristic—because this forms the basis of merit-based selection.

For more on job descriptions and person specifications, see Chapter 14 (page 153).

3. Having position checked

Once a job description and person specification have been constructed, another member of the organisation should check them for consistency, typographical quality and accuracy, and whether the position is presented in a positive and attractive manner. A nurse's decision of whether to apply for a postion often depends entirely on the job description and person specification. It is therefore important that the position is presented in the most positive way.

Nurse managers should ensure that:

▶ the position is comparable with similar positions in the organisation (ensuring that it is not too demanding or complicated compared with others);

▶ the position is correctly classified and complies with any award requirements (statutory employment conditions);

▶ relevant employment conditions and employment awards are fulfilled;

▶ there is an adequate budget to cover the position, and that it is part of the staff plan; and

▶ correct classification grades have been applied (for example, full-time, part-time, permanent, or temporary), and that the number of hours the post-holder will be expected to work in any rostered period is clearly stated.

Finally, in some countries and states, the organisation might be required to determine if there are any available local nurses who should be offered the position before it is advertised.

Key characteristics

In recruiting staff, nurse managers should especially look for the following key characteristics:

• enthusiasm;
• creativity;
• leadership;
• ability to perform under pressure;
• flexibility;
• decision-making;
• the ability to work in a team;
• communication skills;
• business management skills; and
• client advocacy.

4. Advertising the position

Once the job description and person specification have been reviewed and approved, the next step is to inform as many potential candidates as possible that the position is available. The position might be advertised internally (within the organisation) or externally (through professional journals, employment agencies, recruitment firms, government publications, or mainstream advertising on billboards, radio, or television). Advertising can be in print media or electronic media, or through direct contact (for example, by presentations to new graduates).

The choice of the most suitable advertising medium depends on the target group, cost, practicality, schedules, and employer policy. There are advantages and disadvantages associated with all media. For example, many professional journals have specific targeted readerships, but are published only quarterly.

Whichever method of advertising is chosen, attention needs to be given to the wording of the advertisement itself. Nurse managers should remember that they are advertising not only a nursing position, but also the employer. Advertisements should emphasise positive aspects of the organisation, the conditions of employment, staff amenities, and future opportunities for career development.

'Nurse managers should remember that they are advertising not only a nursing position, but also the employer.'

Depending on the organisation's policies, an advertisement usually consists of a brief description of the role's key components, with an emphasis on its attractive components. This should be taken directly from the job description. The advertisement should also describe how applications should be presented and what applicants need to address. Many employers favour the use of standard employment application forms because these help to ensure that candidates provide the information required. The advertisement should also provide details of persons with whom candidates can discuss the position. This must be a person who is readily available and who has a sound understanding of the position.

Advertising

Advertising can be in print media or electronic media, or by direct presentation. All have certain advantages and disadvantages.

This advertising might be conducted through professional journals, employment agencies, recruitment firms, government publications, or mainstream advertising on billboards, radio, or television.

Nurse managers should remember that they are advertising not only a nursing position, but also the employer.

5. Establishing the selection panel

While waiting for responses to the advertising, the organisation should establish a selection panel. Care should be taken to avoid very large panels. For most positions four members is adequate. Selection panels should include:

▶ the responsible line manager (who is usually the chair of the panel);

▶ representatives of groups who most relate to the position (consumers, carers, and staff members who report to the position); and

▶ a peer (someone of the same grade or a person in a similar post).

In establishing the selection panel, consideration should also be given to including external members from other organisations or departments, ensuring a gender balance, and providing a mix of disciplines or staff groups. If members have limited experience on selection panels, it might be necessary to organise training for the selection panel to ensure that all members have a good understanding of the process and skills required.

Skills required of panel members are:

▶ knowledge of the selection process;

▶ maintenance of strict confidentiality;

▶ involvement and agreement with all facets of the selection process;

▶ awareness of all information regarding candidates;

▶ impartiality, fairness, and openness (especially in declaring any potential conflict of interest);

▶ thorough notation of all deliberations;

▶ being prepared to make a minority report if members find themselves dissenting from the majority of the panel; and

▶ knowledge of any relevant legislation, policies, and procedures.

Establishing a selection committee

Selection panels should include:

• the responsible line manager (who is usually the chair of the panel);

• representatives of groups who most relate to the position (consumers, carers, and staff members who report to the position); and

• a peer (someone of the same grade or a person in a similar post).

Consideration should also be given to including external members from other organisations or departments, ensuring a gender balance, and providing a mix of disciplines or staff groups.

6. Shortlisting the candidates

Once all applications have been received, the panel should convene to consider candidates for interview and/or shortlisting. Decisions on which candidates are to be interviewed or shortlisted should be based on information contained in the applications.

This task is made easier and more objective if the panel decides on valid selection criteria *before* looking at the applications. This can be done using the job and person specification as a template—thereby determining what methods the panel will use to measure these criteria.

In shortlisting candidates, the intention should be to include candidates, rather than exclude them. If the panel is unclear whether a particular candidate meets the shortlisting criteria, more information should be sought from that person.

7. Undertaking a selection process

Having shortlisted candidates for a position, the panel should embark on the actual selection. Useful sources of information for assessing the merit of each candidate are:

▶ previous relevant experience as detailed in the person's curriculum vitae, work records, and any available performance reviews (usually the most important criterion);

▶ academic and professional qualifications;

▶ references; and

▶ information from the application process (including written application and interview)—especially evidence that the person has the potential to improve or extend himself or herself in the position.

Most panels interview shortlisted candidates personally, but this is not mandatory. Selection panels might wish to consider the use of presentations, demonstration of practical skills, or other creative means of assessing candidates. Although it is unusual, candidates are occasionally appointed without an interview.

8. Conducting the interview

It is the chair's responsibility to manage the interview process by selecting an appropriate venue, ensuring privacy and comfort and, as far as possible, making the interview a non-threatening experience. The chair should explain the interview process, introduce panel members by name and role, and answer any questions from candidates.

The interview should not be seen as an oral examination that candidates either pass or fail. The interview is essentially a forum for a two-way exchange of information and impressions. It is an opportunity for the potential employer and the candidate to present themselves in the most positive manner. In general, interviews should not exceed 45 minutes in duration, and a few questions from each panel member are adequate.

'The interview should not be seen as an oral examination that candidates either pass or fail . . . it is essentially a two-way exchange of information and impressions.'

The interview should also allow time for the nurse manager and the candidate to clarify any issues or questions about the application or the position. The use of telephone or video-link interviewing is becoming more widespread as technology becomes easier to access. This method is increasingly used in remote areas around the world. Caution should be exercised when using such technologies for only some candidates, because bias can be introduced.

If possible, questions should be open-ended and should give the candidate an opportunity to describe tangible real instances in which he or she has demonstrated competence in key criteria (such as decision-making). In assessing any criterion, the best predictors of success are a recent and long history of achievement in that particular criterion.

Questions should focus on work history, rather than personal matters. If a candidate fails to convince the panel of the reliability of a response, or seems to struggle with a question, a panel member should rephrase the question or ask for additional detail.

At the conclusion of the interview, the chair should ask the candidate if he or she has any questions, and should invite the candidate to make a closing comment.

9. Checking references

References are a valuable source of information for the panel and should always be requested as soon as possible in the selection process. All referees should be contacted for a reference. However, sighting of references requires the candidate's permission. If a candidate does not include his or her current employer as a referee, the omission should be noted and followed up.

In seeking a reference, the selection panel should ask the referee to address specific areas identified by the panel. Many organisations use reference request forms to ensure that references contain sufficient comment and detail. Verbal references, with detailed note-taking by the interviewer, are also acceptable.

10. Making the decision

Provided that decisions about key criteria and the assessment of those criteria have been sound, a decision on the successful candidate is usually relatively simple. In making a selection, panels can use consensus or take a majority decision.

Apart from the selected candidate, the panel should also identify other candidates who could be offered the position if the first-ranked candidate subsequently declines the position. Scoring of criteria can make it easier to rank candidates in terms of merit.

If no suitable candidates emerge from the process, the panel should review the position, the job description and person specification, the selection process, and the advertising process before recommencing.

11. Writing the selection report

At the conclusion of the panel's deliberations, the chair should complete a selection report. There are many acceptable formats, but all should contain:

▶ the exact position to be filled (including its background, history, and conditions);
▶ full details of the selection panel;
▶ the selection criteria used by the panel for shortlisting and final selection;
▶ details of the short-listing procedures and, if applicable, justification for failing to shortlist certain candidates;
▶ details of the shortlisted candidates, and a summary of the assessment of each candidate;
▶ the panel's conclusion and recommendation;
▶ the signature of each panel member, and approval by the delegated authority; and
▶ a retained single copy of all documents associated with the process (with all other documentation that relates to the selection process having been destroyed).

Finally, the completed selection report and recommendation should be authorised by the relevant employer representative. Selection panels seldom have delegated authority to formalise the appointment of the candidate, and the authorisation of the selection process represents a finalisation of the panel's deliberations.

12. Informing the candidates

After the completion of the selection process, the candidates are informed of the outcome. This can be done verbally or in writing, and is the responsibility of the chair of the selection panel. Verbal advice should always be immediately followed by written advice that includes details of any grievance avenues available.

After the selection has been made

Having made the selection, the recruitment process still has several important stages to complete. These include:
- completion of a selection report (which should be formally authorised);
- informing the candidates of the results of the process; and
- inducting the successful candidate.

These important steps are discussed in greater detail in this section of the text.

All candidates should be offered feedback on their application at a later date. Candidates can be quite emotional when informed of the panel's decision and might not fully comprehend feedback provided at the time.

The successful candidate should be notified first. If he or she declines the position, this enables the second-ranked candidate to be approached without revealing that he or she was not the preferred applicant.

13. Inducting the successful candidate

Once any final conditions and a commencement date have been agreed with the successful candidate, a comprehensive induction and orientation program should be instituted. The extent of this process will depend on the individual's previous experience with the organisation, but the successful candidate should be made aware of:

- full details of the job specification to ensure that he or she appreciates areas of immediate and longer-term priority and his or her key responsibilities;
- how the person's performance within the position will be appraised;
- the organisation's role, strategic directions, and philosophy;
- key staff and contacts;
- persons responsible for planning and evaluation of work systems, routines, programs, and clinical care;
- communication methods and channels within the organisation;
- documentation that is available for staff guidance (for example, policy manuals);
- principles of safe work practice and risk minimisation;
- access to available professional development;

- the physical layout of the organisation;
- the procedures for proper use of any equipment;
- established routines and schedules;
- processes of clinical care (including assessment, management planning, involvement of family and others, and documentation); and
- an overview of those who receive care from the organisation.

Retention strategies

There are many reasons for the worldwide shortage of nurses. These include:

- the ageing nursing workforce;
- the negative effects of shift work;
- undesirable award (employment) conditions, particularly low rates of pay;
- poor career paths and lack of variety and stimulation in work;
- heavy workloads, low nursing numbers, and workplace stress;
- limited access to relevant, affordable education;
- an increase in aggression and violence in the workplace;
- increased work choices for women;
- burnout and lack of job satisfaction;
- lack of professional support and supervision;
- undesirable conditions and a lack of amenities (for example, parking, security);
- high physical demands and workplace injury;
- lack of workplace flexibility;
- inadequate recognition and status;
- increasing client acuity and complexity; and
- poor leadership.

In attempting to ameliorate some of these factors and retain staff members, individual nurse managers can adopt the following two strategies:

- adopting a supportive and positive attitude to nurses in general; and
- adopting an individualised approach to staff retention.

Each of these is discussed below.

Attitude to nurses

Because of the interface role they fulfil between individual nurses and the organisation, nurse managers are pivotal in influencing and communicating the organisation's attitude to nurses. As the biggest employee group within health services, nurses consume the largest slice of the budget. In too many organisations, budget pressures result in nurses being seen as an expensive burden, rather than as a valuable resource. This attitude is then demonstrated to nurses in a host of covert and overt negative messages about the value placed on them and the investment in them.

Nurse managers should ensure that nurses feel supported and valued as a vital part of the healthcare team. As Gordon (2002) observed:

'In too many organisations, budget pressures result in nurses being seen as an expensive burden, rather than as a valuable resource.'

> We have never wavered in our support of the nurse at the bedside . . . Through the good times and lean times, we have . . . never, ever cut a nursing position . . . We view nurses as cost avoiders.

Nurse managers who genuinely convey this attitude to their staff and who publicly advocate this view within their organisations at all levels are more successful in retaining their staff.

Two important retention strategies

In the face of a worldwide shortage of nurses, managers can have an important positive effect on staff retention. Two useful strategies to employ are:
- adopting a supportive and positive attitude to nurses in general; and
- adopting an individualised approach to staff retention.

Each of these is discussed in this portion of the text.

An individualised approach

The reasons for nurses remaining in the profession or choosing to leave are as individual as nurses themselves. Although broad retention strategies (across provinces, states, or nations) are useful in planning systemic changes, they are only part of the picture. The nurse manager cannot rely on system-wide responses to nurse retention and cannot assume that 'one size fits all'.

'The nurse manager cannot rely on system-wide responses to nurse retention and cannot assume that "one size fits all".'

Some nurses enjoy the flexibility of shift work, whereas others loathe it. Some nurses choose to work nights, whereas others avoid it. The focus must be on understanding the factors that provide individual nurses with job satisfaction. Retention is not always about benefits and remuneration; in fact, many nurses take a pay cut for a more satisfying job.

Effective nurse managers take time and make an effort to understand the needs of individual nurses, and seek to negotiate arrangements that are suitable to each of them. The key to this individualised approach is flexibility in any work setting. To achieve this, the nurse manager should consider:

◗ scheduling regular meetings with all nurses;
◗ conducting regular staff-satisfaction audits and reviews, and act on exit interviews;
◗ approaching other organisations to find out what they are doing to retain staff;
◗ understanding award and employment conditions to ensure that nurses benefit fully from any provisions that they contain;
◗ enacting clinical-rotation systems and succession-planning systems to provide nurses with variety and career paths;
◗ exploring and communicating professional-development opportunities to nurses (because many are busy and might not be aware of what is currently available to them); and
◗ ensuring, through well-constructed and cogent argument, that the organisation's managers fully understand the real costs of not retaining nurses.

Conclusion

Selecting, recruiting, and retaining talented and motivated nurses is a vital task for any nurse manager. It has a profound effect on the provision of clinical care.

Although there are no 'quick fixes' for the current nursing shortage, there is reason for optimism as government, health services, and the nursing profession increase efforts to attract and keep nurses.

Individual nurse managers can contribute by following the lead of the environmental movement and 'thinking globally and acting locally'.

Chapter 16

Rostering

Cherrie Lowe

Introduction

The roster is one of the most important tools used by nurse managers to plan and manage human resources, and rostering is a complex and demanding function that is often not accorded the attention and respect it requires. Skills for developing rosters are usually learnt on the job, and few nurse managers are educated in the development of effective rosters (Bonner, Beaumont & Smith 1995a).

Effective rosters achieve three main objectives: (i) high-quality patient outcomes; (ii) staff satisfaction; and (iii) financial outcomes within budget parameters.

This chapter:

▶ outlines how changing healthcare environments affect
roster design;

▶ defines rostering objectives and outlines the key elements required to achieve these objectives;

▶ introduces a range of methodologies and describes their relative advantages and disadvantages;

▶ gives a practical example of how to measure the number of labour hours per patient day that a roster pattern will absorb (and guidance on how to estimate associated costs); and

▶ describes the purpose and process of roster re-engineering.

The healthcare environment

Nursing services operate in a changing environment. Some of the major factors producing these changes include:

▶ rapidly changing technology;

▶ an ageing population with an increasing dependence on health care;

▶ a decrease in the average length of stay in acute-care facilities;

▶ an increased dependence on nursing care in hospitals (as measured by patient acuity data); and

▶ an increase in demand for community-based healthcare services.

'A combination of factors has produced a general increase in the daily workload of nursing services.'

This combination of factors has produced a general increase in the daily workload of nursing services.

Nurse managers responsible for nursing services are faced with the additional challenges of tighter healthcare budgets, a global shortage of experienced and competent nurses, more demanding workplace conditions and restraints, and an ageing and less flexible workforce.

In addition, nursing workload peaks, nursing intensity during each episode of care, and the development of specialist trained staff have all been affected by changing circumstances. These include changes in admission and discharge patterns, an increase in the hours of service, more frequent 'day-only' admissions, the use of high-tech equipment, and a decrease in patients' length of stay.

Objectives of roster development

The staff roster is a management tool that is used to plan how and when human resources are utilised. The three main objectives of the process of rostering are:

▶ high-quality patient outcomes (see this chapter, page 179);

▶ staff satisfaction (see this chapter, page 187); and

▶ cost-effectiveness (see this chapter, page 194).

Objectives of roster development

The objectives of roster development are:
* *high-quality patient outcomes* (see this chapter, below);
* *staff satisfaction* (see this chapter, page 187); and
* *cost-effectiveness* (see this chapter, page 194).

These objectives are fundamental to the process of roster development and therefore form the framework for this chapter.

High-quality patient outcomes

Patient outcomes are directly affected by the level of experience, skill, and commitment of the staff. To achieve quality patient outcomes the roster must provide:

▶ adequate clinical hours for each shift to complete care (both direct and indirect);

▶ an appropriate range of shift lengths and starting times to ensure that peak activity periods are covered and that staff breaks are accommodated; and

▶ an appropriate staff skill mix for each shift to ensure patient needs are met.

Each of these is discussed below.

Adequate clinical hours

Patient acuity data are used to ensure that adequate clinical hours are allowed for each shift to complete direct and indirect care. Patient acuity is measured by using a patient nurse dependency system which estimates the level of nursing intensity required. It is necessary to have access to historic patient acuity trends (Bonner, Beaumont & Smith 1995b).

Measures of patient acuity identify the hours required for patient care for each shift. Patient acuity is therefore measured in hours per patient day (HPPD). It has been demonstrated that acuity (that is, nursing intensity required for care) varies on certain days and certain months, regardless of occupancy.

By trending patient acuity over a period of time an acuity profile can be developed. This profile can be weekly, fortnightly, or monthly—depending on the cyclical patterns of scheduled operating lists, programs, clinics, or services. Computerised acuity systems measure the average hours required for care for the evening, day, and night shift for each day and generate a range of reports that can be used for roster development.

An example of a ward acuity profile is demonstrated in Figure 16.1 (page 180). This illustrates a roster re-engineering report produced by a computerised acuity system. This report is used as a roster design sheet. It provides ward managers with acuity data displayed as total nursing hours required for each shift and facilitates the development of a roster pattern that will indicate shift lengths and start and finish times.

Ward roster re-engineering report—clinical hours required

Rostered shift
Average hours required (measured by patient dependency)

Ward: [name/number/description of ward] Period of: [month/year to month/year]

Shift	Monday	Tuesday	Wednesday	Thursday	Friday	Saturday	Sunday
EARLY 0700–1530	RNs, RMs / Ens / OTH	RNs, RMs / Ens / OTH	RNs, RMs / Ens / OTH	RNs, RMs / Ens / OTH	RNs, RMs / Ens / OTH	RNs, RMs / Ens / OTH	RNs, RMs / Ens / OTH
	Av. hrs req: 44:35 FTE: (5.5) 5.57	Av. hrs req: 46:56 FTE: (5.5) 5.87	Av. hrs req: 50:15 FTE: (6) 6.28	Av. hrs req: 46:45 FTE: (5.5) 5.84	Av. hrs req: 49:04 FTE: (6) 6.13	Av. hrs req: 44:17 FTE: (5.5) 5.53	Av. hrs req: 40:13 FTE: (5) 5.03
LATE 1430–2300	RNs, RMs / Ens / OTH	RNs, RMs / Ens / OTH	RNs, RMs / Ens / OTH	RNs, RMs / Ens / OTH	RNs, RMs / Ens / OTH	RNs, RMs / Ens / OTH	RNs, RMs / Ens / OTH
	Av. hrs req: 32:39 FTE: (4) 4.08	Av. hrs req: 39:46 FTE: (4.5) 4.97	Av. hrs req: 39:01 FTE: (4.5) 4.88	Av. hrs req: 38:03 FTE: (4.5) 4.76	Av. hrs req: 38:00 FTE: (4.5) 4.75	Av. hrs req: 31:54 FTE: (4) 3.99	Av. hrs req: 31:57 FTE: (4) 3.99
NIGHT 2245–0700	RNs, RMs / Ens / OTH	RNs, RMs / Ens / OTH	RNs, RMs / Ens / OTH	RNs, RMs / Ens / OTH	RNs, RMs / Ens / OTH	RNs, RMs / Ens / OTH	RNs, RMs / Ens / OTH
	Av. hrs req: 18:08 FTE: (2) 2.27	Av. hrs req: 26:40 FTE: (3) 3.33	Av. hrs req: 23:32 FTE: (3) 2.57	Av. hrs req: 25:31 FTE: (3) 3.11	Av. hrs req: 21:05 FTE: (3) 2.64	Av. hrs req: 19:50 FTE: (2) 2.48	Av. hrs req: 19:13 FTE: (2) 2.40
	Av. hrs req: 95:22 FTE: 11.92	Av. hrs req: 113:22 FTE: 14.17	Av. hrs req: 112:48 FTE: 11.92	Av. hrs req: 110:19 FTE: 11.92	Av. hrs req: 108:10 FTE: 11.92	Av. hrs req: 96:01 FTE: 11.92	Av. hrs req: 91:23 FTE: 11.92

Notes: (i) This report identifies the average required hours for each shift on each day of the week for the selected period.
(ii) The report facilitates the development of a roster profile based on acuity trends. FTE calculated on 8-hr shifts.
(iii) The built-in unpredicted value of 12½% has not been included in the day and evening shift totals.

Figure 16.1 Ward roster re-engineering report
© Trend Care Systems Pty Ltd, published with permission

High-quality patient outcomes

Patient outcomes are directly affected by the level of experience, skill, and commitment of the staff. To achieve quality patient outcomes the roster must provide:
- adequate clinical hours for each shift to complete care (both direct and indirect);
- an appropriate range of shift lengths and starting times to ensure that peak activity periods are covered and that staff breaks are accommodated; and
- an appropriate staff skill mix for each shift to ensure patient needs are met.

Each of these issues is discussed in this section of the text.

Appropriate range of shift lengths and starting times

To ensure that peak activity periods are covered and that staff breaks are accommodated, an appropriate range of shift lengths and starting times is required. This is obtained from a consideration of departmental activity.

Regular patient-care activity trends generate increased workload at specific times within a shift. Examples include admission and discharge trends, elective surgery, patient transfer patterns, routine patient-care activities, doctors' rounds, and routine clinics or services.

It is important to give careful consideration to the time at which patient activities start and finish, and the effect that they have on the absorption of resources.

'Careful consideration should be given to the time at which patient activities start and finish, and the effect that they have on the absorption of resources.'

An analysis of ward work studies reveals that workload usually peaks in the first half of the morning shift. Additional nursing hours should therefore be provided during the first four hours of this shift. The workload in the afternoon peaks in the middle of the shift (between 1700 hrs and 2100 hrs). During this peak period nurses also require a meal break, and this increases the workload for those nurses who remain on the ward if additional hours are not rostered for this period. The peak activity period for the night shift falls during the last two hours of the shift when patients are usually awake. These peaks and troughs in workload are clearly depicted in Figure 16.2 (page 182).

The most effective method of managing the workload during peak activity times is to utilise short shifts. Part-time staff can be routinely rostered on short shifts—for example, short 4-hour day shift (0700 hrs to 1100 hrs) and short 4-hour evening shift (1700 hrs to 2100 hrs).

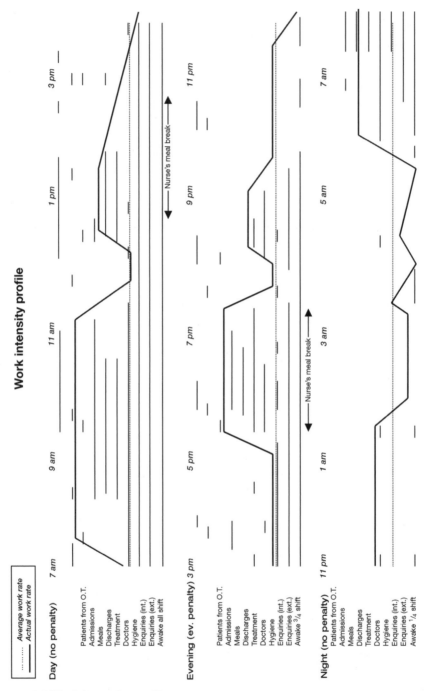

Work intensity profile

Day (no penalty)

Evening (ev. penalty)

Night (no penalty)

Figure 16.2 Work intensity profile
© Trend Care Systems Pty Ltd, published with permission

The night duty workload during peak activity time is most effectively managed by rostering one or two day shifts to start 1–2 hours earlier than the normal day shift—thus providing additional work hours for the last one or two hours of the shift.

If these peak activity periods are not accommodated nurses will become fatigued and patient-care activities will not be completed—thus compromising patient care. The effect of this is magnified when unpredicted activity occurs in the second half of the shift, with nurses being unable to complete their shifts on time. Rostering staggered full shifts also relieves the workload during these peak periods, but will be less financially effective.

> 'If peak activity periods are not accommodated nurses will become fatigued—thus compromising patient care.'

In critical-care areas, peaks and troughs are usually not as consistent on a shift-by-shift basis. A creative combination of long shifts and short shifts usually produces the required roster objectives. The use of 12-hour shifts can be effective in critical-care units in achieving roster objectives. Staff members working in critical-care areas have reported high levels of satisfaction with these shifts. To achieve patient continuity, staff satisfaction, and cost-efficiency, the following principles apply:

▶ the number of 12-hour shifts utilised should be limited to 60–70% of rostered hours;

▶ 12-hour shifts should make up the core staffing and should be complemented by a mix of 8-hour, 6-hour, and 4-hour shifts;

▶ a maximum of three 12-hour shifts should be worked in a week by any one nurse; and

▶ nurses working three 12-hour shifts in a week should have their shifts rostered together and days off not split (because work fatigue is minimised when days off are grouped together).

The roster profiles shown in Figure 16.3 (page 184) demonstrate two different roster patterns for an evening shift which, by acuity, requires 40 hours of care. It is evident that the profile shown as 'Option B' best matches the peaks and troughs in workload for the shift and would therefore be most likely to achieve objectives.

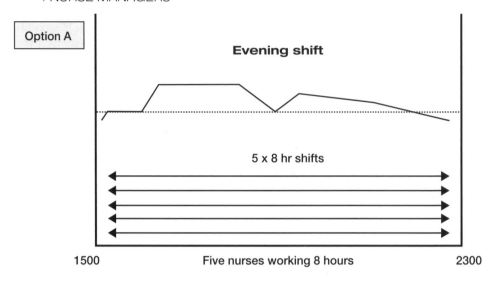

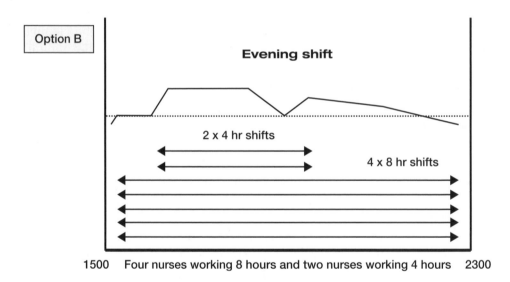

Figure 16.3 Rostering to peaks and troughs in workload
© Trend Care Systems Pty Ltd, published with permission

Appropriate staff skill mix

To provide the right skill mix for each shift, managers must be aware of the type of work that has to be done. Consideration must be given to case mix within the ward, average patient length of stay, skill level and scope of practice of staff, and the model of care delivery. Work studies demonstrate that a greater proportion of enrolled nurses and non-licensed carers can be utilised in non-critical care areas. There is less opportunity to use such staff in wards with low acuity, short length of stay, and rapid turnover.

Figure 16.4 (below) demonstrates the type of work conducted by nursing staff in an orthopaedic ward. Figure 16.5 (page 186) demonstrates the type of work in a urology ward. These demonstrate that the staff skill mix required for acute wards varies according to the case mix and length of stay. The skill mix required also varies according to the shift. A higher proportion of enrolled nurses and nursing-support staff can be used on the day shift—in which a higher concentration of basic patient care and related environmental work occurs.

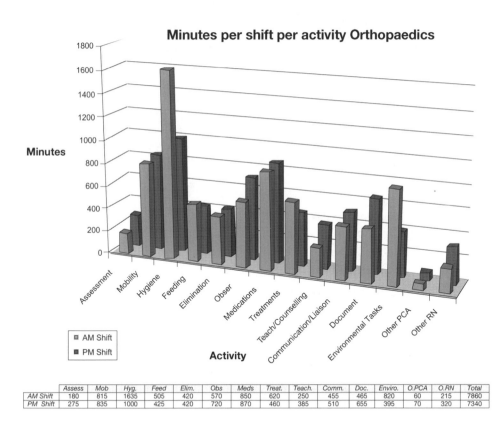

	Assess	Mob	Hyg.	Feed	Elim.	Obs	Meds	Treat.	Teach.	Comm.	Doc.	Enviro.	O.PCA	O.RN	Total
AM Shift	180	815	1635	505	420	570	850	620	250	455	465	820	60	215	7860
PM Shift	275	835	1000	425	420	720	870	460	385	510	655	395	70	320	7340

Figure 16.4 Orthopaedic work profile

© Trend Care Systems Pty Ltd, published with permission

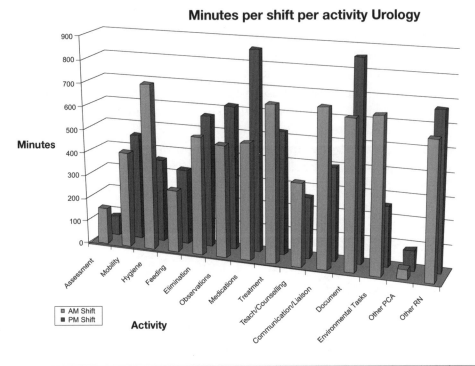

	Assess	Mob	Hyg.	Feed	Elim.	Obs	Meds	Treat.	Teach.	Comm.	Doc.	Enviro.	O.PCA	O.RN	Total
AM Shift	155	410	710	265	505	480	500	670	355	675	640	660	45	585	6655
PM Shift	85	460	360	325	570	620	864	530	260	400	861	260	85	675	6365

Figure 16.5 Urology work profile

© Trend Care Systems Pty Ltd, published with permission

The skill mix should be carefully balanced to ensure that:
▶ patient safety is not compromised;
▶ staff members complete work that lies within their scope of practice;
▶ staff members receive fair and equitable workloads;
▶ there is adequate orientation and supervision for students, novices, and staff members who are new to the environment;
▶ there is a balance between hands-on clinical hours and non-clinical hours;
▶ the proportion of registered nurses to enrolled nurses suits the case mix and the type of work in the ward; and
▶ the level of support staff is proportional to the amount of work available relative to the staff's scope of practice.

If a roster is to provide human resources appropriately over a period of time, it is critical that the creator of that roster is fully aware of all activities occurring during that period. The type and volume of work in a department can be identified by conducting a work study. This involves staff members completing a form for each shift that they work over a one-month period. An appropriate roster skill mix can then be developed. Figure 16.6 (page 188) is a sample of a work study form used to identify work.

'It is critical that the creator of a roster is fully aware of all activities that occur.'

To match clinical work requirements to nursing staff skills, it is essential that the skill level of each nurse be evaluated and that nurses be identified as having particular skill levels. Nursing skill levels can be defined as:

▶ team leader (able to be in charge on a shift);
▶ competent (requires no direct supervision);
▶ advanced beginner (requires guidance in complex situations); and
▶ novice (new practitioner requiring some supervision and guidance).

If each nurse is rated at a level of competence, some automated roster systems can then generate the best skill mix from the nurses available. If set parameters for staffing are not met, the system alerts the user.

If the model of care used to deliver patient care is *primary nursing* or *patient allocation to individual nurses*, the roster will require a skill mix of nurses who are all at a competent level and above. If the model of care is *patient allocation with team nursing*, a range of nurse levels and nursing support staff can be incorporated into the roster.

Staff satisfaction

Importance of staff satisfaction

The second of the objectives of roster development noted on page 178 was *staff satisfaction*. The type and number of shifts allocated to staff members can have a substantial effect on staff satisfaction because these shifts affect:

▶ the economic circumstances of staff members;
▶ the time and energy spent with families and in activities other than work;
▶ the health of staff members;
▶ the degree of satisfaction achieved from work; and
▶ opportunities to learn and develop.

As a result of increasing workplace democracy staff members have more input into their roster design, and are generally better protected and provided for by workplace rules. Before posting a roster, the nurse manager responsible for that

Work Study Data Collection Instrument

Hospital: .... RN: .... Start Time: .... Day of Week: ....

Ward: .... Shift: .... Finish Time: .... Date: ....

Ward Management

Bed management	✓	Resource issues and data entry	✓	Teaching and support staff	✓
Allocating beds for admissions		Calling in staff to work		Demonstrating skills	
Moving patients		Liaising with hospital coordinator		Supervising practice	
		Reviewing trend care		Emotionally supporting staff	
		Updating trend care		Evaluating competence	
		Organising meal relief		Orientating new staff	
		Making roster changes			
		Data entry excluding trend care and all of the above			
				Time	Hrs	Min

Advanced Clinical Activities

Doctors' rounds	✓	Discharge planning	✓	Assessments	✓	Teaching and counselling	✓	Communicating and liaising	✓	Documentation	✓
Attending doctor rounds (routine)		Organising medication		Patient history		Patient teaching		Taking doctor phone calls		Patient progress reports	
Attending teaching rounds		Contacting relatives		Risk assessments • falls • pressure areas • nutrition • discharge		Patient counselling		Taking relative calls		Care plans and clinical pathways	
		Organising transport				Relative teaching		Liaising with AHP		Discharge summaries	
		Organising community support				Relative counselling		Liaising with doctors		Incident reports	
				Wound assessment				Managing complaints			
				HONOS				Contacting clergy			
				BARTELLS				Liaising with other departments			
				FIMS				Liaising with other services			
									Time	Hrs	Min

N.B. Activities not accounted for on this form should be documented in the most appropriate column.

Figure 16.6 Work study data collection form

© Trend Care Systems Pty Ltd, published with permission

Word Study Data Collection Instrument (cont.)

Hospital: ....
Ward: ....
RN: ....
Shift: ....
Start Time: .... Day of Week ....
Finish Time: .... Date ....

Technical Activities

Observations	✓	Medications	✓	Treatment	✓
Routine obs		Oral		Dressing	
Post-op obs		Injections		Removal of tubes and drains	
ICC obs		Infusions		Pre-op preps	
Behavioural		Topical		Insertion of IDC, IV, NG	
BSLs		Rectal/vaginal		Assisting with procedures	
Post procedure		TPN		Dialysis	
		Chemotherapy			
				Time ___ Hrs ___ Min	

Patient Activities of Daily Living

Mobility	✓	Hygiene	✓	Feeding	✓	Elimination	✓	Environmental tasks	✓	Other (describe)	✓
Patient assist to toilet		Assist with shower		Main meal feed		Assist with toileting		Cleaning beds			
Patient assist to bathroom		Assist with bath		Diet ordering		Giving and taking pans and urinals		Cleaning room			
Patient assist with exercise		Bed bath		NG feeds		Emptying IDC		Making beds			
Assist with physio		Face and hands wash				Stoma care		Tidying bathrooms			
Applying CPM machine		Mouth care						Cleaning and tidying pan and treatment utility rooms			
Applying traction		Shave									
Re-position patient								Tidying office			
Pressure area care								Making charts			
								Transporting patients to and from OT, X-ray, etc.			
								Emptying linen skips			
						Time ___ Hrs ___ Min		Time ___ Hrs ___ Min		Time ___ Hrs ___ Min	

Overtime Worked: ___ hrs ___ mins   Meal Break Taken ☐ Yes ☐ No   If "No", reason: _____

TrendCare Actual Required Hrs: _____

TrendCare Actual Clinical Hrs: _____

roster is obliged by law to ensure that all workplace rules and occupational health-and-safety regulations are complied with.

Roster flexibility

To minimise staff fatigue during periods of high absenteeism, more flexible rosters can be achieved by:

- maintaining a mix of permanent full-time and permanent part-time staff members;
- rostering 4-hour shifts to permanent part-time staff (with these shifts being extended if necessary);
- utilising a range of long (12-hr and 10-hr) shifts in combination with short (8-hr, 6-hr, and 4-hr) shifts;
- establishing a *pool roster* whereby permanent full-time and part-time staff members are rostered shifts but are not attached to any ward—being placed on a shift-by-shift basis;
- retaining a group of casual employees;
- establishing working relationships with nursing agencies;
- developing systems that accommodate roster requests and shift changes after roster development; and
- establishing systems such as *time off in lieu*, *banked hours*, and *flex time*.

Involving staff in rostering

If nursing staff are to be involved in roster development they must be educated in workplace rules, occupational health-and-safety requirements, and policies relating to roster requests, annual leave, rostered days off, and so on. The competence level of each nurse and the skill mix profile for each shift must also be shared with staff. Nurses should also be made aware of the nursing intensity required for patient care (measured by acuity for each shift) and peaks and troughs in workload. Financial outcome targets relating to ward salaries should also be known to staff. Finally, requirements for staff training and attendance at meetings should be known to all staff members.

Request-focus rostering

The most common method of rostering is request-focus rostering. This method attempts to accommodate as many staff requests as possible and involves developing a roster 'from the ground up' each time. The method is time-consuming and is best generated by computerised roster systems.

The most common staff complaint related to this model is that some staff members are thought to be favoured. Other staff members find themselves receiving left-over shifts after the favoured staff members have had their requests met.

The advantages and disadvantages of request-focus rostering are listed in the Box below.

'The most common complaint about request-focus rostering is that some staff members are thought to be favoured.'

In summary, this method requires nurse managers to invest significant time to meeting staff requests, providing an adequate skill mix for each shift, and obtaining a cost-effective staffing outcome.

Request-focus rostering: advantages and disadvantages

Advantages

The *advantages* of request-focus rostering are:
- the specific needs of most staff members can usually be met;
- it is possible to incorporate a range of shift lengths and start and finish times;
- the roster can be generated by a computerised rostering system; and
- staff members who have requests accommodated are satisfied.

Disadvantages

The *disadvantages* of the method are:
- it is a time-consuming process (taking 6–8 hours);
- workplace rules, occupational health-and-safety requirements, and ward-rostering policies are often compromised;
- some staff members feel disadvantaged;
- it is difficult to obtain optimum skill mix from the staff available while also accommodating all staff requests; and
- the method cannot easily accommodate self-rostering.

Cyclical rotating rosters

This method has pre-set roster patterns developed around workplace rules, occupational health-and-safety requirements, and organisational policies. Each line represents a nurse roster and is given a unique number and skill level. The allocation of nurses to the set roster patterns can be done on a fortnightly, monthly, six-weekly, or two-monthly basis by the nurse manager or by the nurses themselves using self-rostering concepts. This method of rostering can be very popular when implemented with skill and equity.

The advantages and disadvantages of cyclical rotating rostering are listed in the Box on page 192.

Cyclical rotating rostering: advantages and disadvantages

Advantages

The *advantages* of cyclical rotating rostering are:
- workplace rules, occupational safety requirements, and ward-rostering policies are easily incorporated and maintained;
- staff members are able to predict their work pattern in advance;
- the method can be accommodated on simple spreadsheets or sophisticated roster systems;
- roster development time is short;
- it is possible to optimise shift skill mix from available resources;
- a fair and equitable shift distribution is achieved;
- the method can accommodate self-rostering concepts; and
- shifts can be swapped within the finalised roster.

Disadvantages

The *disadvantages* of the method are:
- the roster usually takes 6–8 hours to complete;
- multiple requests within a week might not be accommodated easily;
- many nursing staff members reject this rigid process; and
- some staff members become inflexible and resist moving from one cycle to another to accommodate others.

Self-rostering

During the past decade or so, the concept of self-rostering has become popular. The main objective of this method is to increase staff satisfaction and to attract and retain skilled nursing staff (Vetter, Felice & Ingersoll 2001). If this method is implemented, it is critical that all nurses concerned fully understand the rules of rostering, the outcome objectives for the ward, and the minimum requirements for staffing each shift for each day of the week.

'The main objective of self-rostering is to increase staff satisfaction and to attract and retain skilled nursing staff.'

The advantages and disadvantages of self-rostering are listed in the Box on page 193.

Self-rostering works best in units in which there is a variety of personal circumstances among staff members, and in which staff members have different preferences about work patterns (Fudge 2001).

Self-rostering: advantages and disadvantages

Advantages

The *advantages* of self-rostering are;
- improved staff understanding of rostering;
- staff having more control over hours worked;
- improved flexibility if staff members are prepared to work additional shifts, change starting times, and so on;
- improved staff satisfaction and reduced absenteeism;
- ability to match staff roster needs with ward staffing needs;
- staff being able to plan out-of-work activities more easily; and
- encouragement of teamwork.

Disadvantages

The *disadvantages* of the method are:
- it requires set protocols and significant staff education;
- it can be difficult matching ward requirements and rules to staff needs;
- workplace rules and occupational health-and-safety requirements can be compromised;
- it requires regular staff satisfaction review;
- some staff members end up with only left-over shifts;
- it can produce additional work for the unit manager if staff members ignore rules;
- there can be problems with staff members meeting the deadline for posting the roster;
- it requires up to four hours of management time to adjust the roster so that it meets all requirements; and
- nurses can become fatigued when they select shifts for social reasons and fail to consider work fatigue.

Evaluating the suitability of rosters

A roster should be regularly evaluated to assess its suitability to the staff and its effectiveness in achieving roster objectives. Rosters plan the working life of people, and their feedback is therefore critical. Staff satisfaction surveys, performance reviews, staff exit interviews or questionnaires can be used for feedback. The nurse manager should ascertain if the roster:
- meets staff needs;
- provides adequate staffing numbers;
- provides an adequate skill mix;
- matches workload peaks and troughs;
- provides an equitable mix of shifts;

▶ provides an adequate skill mix so that novice practitioners, new staff members, and students are appropriately supported; and

▶ provides opportunity for staff professional development.

Other indicators of roster suitability include:

▶ patient outcomes (for example, the incidence of adverse events);

▶ sick leave rates;

▶ staff deployment rates;

▶ staff turnover rates; and

▶ efficiency outcomes related to budget.

Ongoing evaluation should be conducted to measure the degree to which the roster meets workload demand, provides equitable treatment for all staff, meets staff personal preferences, and satisfies occupational health-and-safety requirements. Attention should also be paid to whether the roster complies with industrial and legal requirements, minimises staff fatigue, and maximises efficient use of resources.

Cost-effectiveness
Difficulties with budgets

The third of the objectives of roster development noted on page 178 was *cost-effectiveness*. Budgetary restrictions place enormous pressures on nurse managers who are required to provide consistent quality care to a growing number of more complex patients.

'Budgetary restrictions place enormous pressures on nurse managers in providing consistent quality care to a growing number of more complex patients.'

Nurse managers are often presented with a budget target which they have not been involved in developing. This target is usually presented either as a financial figure or as a certain number of labour hours. The latter is usually expressed as a certain number of hours per patient per day (HPPD) (see this chapter, page 179).

Data and information required

To achieve a pre-set target budget the nurse manager must clarify exactly what is included in the budgeted target. This involves a clarification of the average cost per productive hour for each staff type and all 'on costs' that are included in the target (for example, penalty rates, superannuation, and so on). The manager must also ascertain the projected patient throughput for the next

12-month period, and identify peaks and troughs in workload according to patient dependency data. From this information the manager can decide on a suitable staff mix.

It will be necessary to collect retrospective data on absenteeism rates for the past 12 months and identify the number of hours required per month for staff to attend meetings. The manager must also calculate the hours required for training and orientation and the number of supernumerary hours required for ward supervision on the evening and weekend shifts.

The manager must also calculate casual and agency usage as a percentage of total clinical hours worked, identify the number of hours required per month for clerical, orderly, and other support staff, and ascertain the number of nurse-management hours required.

Calculations

Using retrospective acuity data a roster profile can be established (see Figure 16.1, page 180). To establish the average daily clinical hours per patient day (HPPD) from a roster profile, the following steps should be taken.

1. Total the average number of full-time equivalent shifts rostered for each shift of the week (A) shifts.

2. Calculate the average hours per week (A x 8) hours.

3. Calculate the average hours per day (B) by dividing the weekly number (obtained in point 2) by 7. $\dfrac{(a \times 8)}{7}$

4. Calculate the average number of patients per day (C).

5. Calculate the average number of hours per patient per day by dividing B by C. This gives the HPPD. $\dfrac{B}{C}$

6. Allow for casual or agency hours (for example, 10%) for sick leave and unpredictable peaks in workloads.

7. Calculate total HPPD by adding the number obtained at Step 5 to the number obtained at Step 6.

   Table 16.1 (page 196) shows an example of such a calculation.

   Having calculated the HPPD, the nurse manager can then calculate the cost of rostered clinical hours. By assigning the appropriate monetary value to the HPPD (in terms of various staff members' salaries per hour), the total cost of the roster can be calculated on a daily, monthly, or annual basis.

Table 16.1 Calculation of HPPD

Step	Example
1. Total the average number of full-time equivalent (FTE) shifts rostered for each shift of the week (A) shifts.	87.5 FTE
2. Calculate the average hours per week (A x 8) hours	700 hours
3. Calculate the average hours per day (B) by dividing the weekly number (obtained in Step 2) by 7.	100 hours
4. Calculate the average number of patients per day (C).	26 patients
5. Calculate the average number of hours per patient per day by dividing B by C. This gives the HPPD.	3.85 HPPD
6. Allow casual or agency hours (for example, 10%) for sick leave and unpredictable peaks in workloads.	0.38 HPPD
7. Calculate total HPPD by adding the number obtained at Step 5 to the number obtained at Step 6.	4.23 HPPD (3.85 + 0.38)

Author's creation

Roster re-engineering

It has been found from patient acuity data that certain wards require higher nursing hours per patient per day than do other wards. This explains why some surgical wards of the same size and occupancy require more nursing hours and have higher costs.

If there is a change in the type of patients or the type of treatment in a given ward or unit, the required resources also change. If rosters are to reflect the altered ward activity, acuity, and skill mix requirements, they must change as the case mix, length of stay, or treatment methods change. This process is known as *roster re-engineering*.

Roster re-engineering should be undertaken on an annual basis. The worksheet shown in Figure 16.2 (page 182) was generated by a computerised acuity/patient dependency system for the general purpose of roster re-engineering.

Indications for initiating roster re-engineering include:
- introduction of new services;
- change in ward case mix;
- change in surgical or treatment activity;
- significant decrease in average length of stay;
- change in patient acuity;

▶ introduction of a new staff skill mix; and

▶ need to improve efficiency.

The benefits of roster-re-engineering include: (i) more timely response to patients' needs; (ii) improved morale; (iii) decreased fatigue; (iv) improved satisfaction; and (v) more efficient utilisation of human resources.

Conclusion

The outcomes of rostering are critical to the operation of any healthcare service, and the roster should be recognised by nurse managers as the most important human-resource management tool at their disposal.

Application of the principles and techniques outlined in this chapter will enable nurse managers to maximise the benefits to staff and patients alike in this critical aspect of nurse management.

'The roster should be recognised by nurse managers as the most important human-resource management tool at their disposal.'

Chapter 17

Budgeting

Rita Gan

Introduction

A budget is a formalised planning tool used by management to compare expected revenues with expected expenses for the year (Finkler & Kovner 2000). The objective of budgeting is to maximise organisational resources to meet short-term and long-term goals (Marquis & Huston 2003). A budget can therefore be understood as a written financial plan that aims to control resources (Huber 2000).

The preparation of a budget ensures that an organisation's managers plan ahead and forecast the future—anticipating changes that will affect the organisation so that action plans can be formulated accordingly. For example, a decreasing birth rate is likely to lead to decreased patient days in the maternity wards. A budget can (and should) be used by

'A budget can motivate managers and their staff to work positively to meet their organisation's goals.'

managers to motivate themselves and their staff to work positively to meet their organisation's goals.

A business plan is formulated for the coming year. This involves the key management staff members coming together to review the organisation's performance in terms of the achievement of key performance indicators in financial terms and/or in terms of other value-added indicators (such as customer service satisfaction). A SWOT (strengths, weaknesses, obstacles, and threats) analysis can be used to evaluate an organisation. From such an evaluation, critical success factors can be drawn. Figure 17.1 (below) illustrates a framework for a business plan.

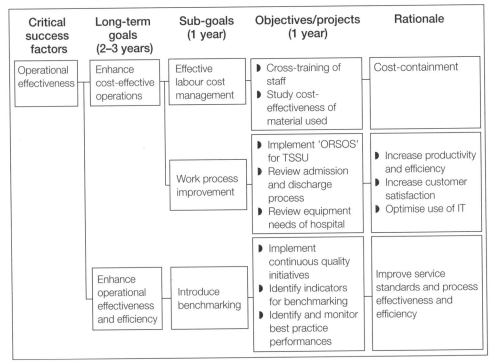

Figure 17.1 Example of a business plan framework
Author's creation, adapted from Parkway Group Healthcare, Singapore

Long-term and short-term goals and objectives are then set. These organisation-wide goals and objectives are then cascaded down to individual divisions and departments. Members of the nursing division, one of the largest divisions in any healthcare setting, will get together to formulate their goals and objectives for the year. This involves the participation of nurse executives and managers at various levels. Which members of the nursing staff are involved in the budget process depends on the particular organisation. Some organisations have a centralised process, whereas others adopt a professional practice model in which the role of individuals is crucial for the achievement of a department's goals, objectives, and budget plan. Whichever model is adopted, the day-to-day monitoring and control of the budget require commitment from each individual staff member. The budget plan should therefore be made known to individual staff members, and their input obtained, to ensure greater ownership and accountability on the part of all staff members.

> 'The budget plan should be made known to individual staff members to ensure greater ownership and accountability on the part of all staff members.'

Budgeting concepts in health care

There are many terms used in budgeting. Some of these are general terms that are used in a variety of budgetary settings. Others are more specific to healthcare settings. Table 17.1 (page 202) provides a list of some of the more commonly used terms, together with a brief explanation of the meaning of each.

Types of budgets

In health care, nurse managers are involved in three types of budgets (Marrelli 1997). These are *capital budgets*, *operating budgets*, and *personnel budgets*. Each of these is discussed below.

Capital budgets

A *capital budget* is a plan that outlines the forecasted purchase of large, fixed assets, equipment that depreciates, buildings, and renovation work. Depreciation is the amount or cost of an asset attributed to a certain operating period. The finance department will generate a payback analysis before approving such budget items.

Capital assets are usually purchased to replace older items of a similar nature, to improve quality of care, or to provide a new service or expansion of the facility. Capital budget items are referred to as *capital assets*, *long-term investments*, *capital investments*, or *capital acquisitions* (Finkler & Kovner 2000; Marquis & Huston 2003). If an item is to be included in a capital budget, most organisations designate a minimum cost requirement.

Table 17.1 Budgeting concepts in health care

Concept	Description
Assets	Organisation's resources that have a dollar value (for example, personal computers)
Budget	A planning document used by a department or organisation to forecast revenues and expenses
Capital budget	A plan for the acquisition of buildings and equipment that will be used for greater than one year beyond the year of acquisition
Casemix	Type of patients served by a healthcare institution or hospital; includes patient-related variables such as diagnosis, personal characteristics, and patterns of treatment
Cost centre	A revenue-producing or non-revenue-producing department assigned responsibility for costs in part of an organisation
DRGs	Diagnosis-related groups A classification system to control the cost of health care by assigning a cost per diagnostic catergory; includes all services provided
Expenses	Costs of assets or services needed for the provision of patient care and generation of revenue
Fiscal year	A one-year period defined for financial purposes; it can start at any point during a calendar year
Fixed costs	Costs that do not vary according to volume (for example, rental or contract services fees)
Liabilities	The legal financial obligations an organisation has to external parties (that is, money owed)
Operating budget	An annual plan of revenues and expenses for an organistion over a period of one year
Unit of service	The basic measure of an item being produced by an organisation (for example, patient days, number of operations, etc.)
Variable costs	Costs that vary in relation to volume. Variable expenses can be controllable or non-controllable Controllable variable expenses can be controlled by the manager (for example, the number of nurses working on a certain shift and their skill mix) Non-controllable variable expenses include equipment depreciation costs and the number and type of supplies used by patients in an emergency

Author's creation

To begin a capital budget plan, a nurse manager must develop a proposal for investments, and justification for acquiring them. Justification of capital requests includes a description of the item, its costs, and its impact on operating expenses and revenues. The evaluation of capital budget requests should take into account both the quantitative benefits and the qualitative benefits that an asset will provide to the organisation and its customers. However, not all assets are evaluated on a profit basis; some items improve productivity and efficiency (for example, new computer software for staff scheduling), whereas other assets (such as a human patient simulator) improve patient safety and clinical quality.

> 'Some assets improve productivity and efficiency; other assets improve patient safety and clinical quality.'

Table 17.2 shows an example of a capital budget request worksheet in a hospital.

Table 17.2 Example of capital budget request sheet

Type	Quantity	Description	Unit cost	Priority	Depreciation per month	Justification
Replacement	1	IV infusion pump	$6 000	1	$100	Current pump not functioning; has exhausted life span of 5 years
Replacement	1	Portable HP defibrillator	$8 000	1	$150	Need to upgrade current defibrillator to semi-automatic, biphasic model
New	1	Personal computer with CD-Rom and office software	$2 000	2	$50	For nursing staff development and admin tasks by unit manager
Total			$16 000			

Author's creation

Operating budgets

An *operating budget* is a plan for the day-to-day operating revenues and expenses of the organisation. It includes fixed costs—for example, service contracts for maintenance of medical or office equipment, medical and non-medical supplies, electricity costs, minor equipment, and education and training expenses. The operating budget forecasts revenue by estimating the number of patient days, average lengths of stay, and units of service. A unit of service is the measurement of the work performed by the cost centre. Workload can be measured in different ways, such as the number of patient visits, deliveries, treatments, or surgical procedures. Units of service provide a basis for both revenue and expense calculations for the coming year.

The responsibility for forecasting patient days and patient revenue falls on a marketing or sales department in a for-profit healthcare organisation. In recent years however, nurse managers have been expected to become more concerned about revenue (Finkler & Kovner 2000). With the emergence of new funding arrangements based on diagnostic groups and designated therapeutic services (such as 'casemix'), it is possible to charge patients for nursing each day, based on patient classification.

> 'In recent years nurse managers have been expected to become more concerned about revenue.'

Personnel budgets

Because healthcare organisations are labour-intensive, the *personnel budget* is the largest component of the operating budget (Grohar-Murray & DiCroce 2003; Marquis & Huston 2003).

A personnel or full-time equivalent (FTE) budget forecasts the actual staffing needs of a department. Staffing requirements include nursing staff of various skill levels and competency, and clerical and housekeeping staff. There is no universal standard for staffing levels. Each healthcare facility has its own unique mix of services, types of patients, and philosophy on the appropriate provision of care. An FTE is equal to one person working 8 hours a day, 5 or 6 days a week, 52 weeks a year. It can be expressed as 1.0 (full-time) or 0.5 (part-time). One FTE does not necessary refer to one person—it can be made up of two or three persons providing workload hours to represent one full-time shift (Marrelli 1997). In calculating staffing expenses, costs must be allocated for both productive and non-productive hours. Non-productive hours include sick leave, holidays, and time spent in educational seminars. A manager needs to establish the type and number of positions required per shift, because these will determine labour costs (for example, base salaries, benefits, bonuses, overtime hours, and other differentials).

The standard formula for calculating nursing care hours (NCH) per patient day (PPD) is shown below.

NCH/PPD = nursing hours worked in 24 hours/patient census

Productivity in healthcare involves a measurement to quantify the effectiveness of staff (Marrelli 1997). The introduction of management engineers who perform time-and-motion studies has resulted in the determination of nursing-care standards. All activities of patient care are examined and quantified into the number of nursing hours. Nursing hours are then converted into FTEs and appropriate skills mix. Management engineers work closely with nurse managers in a consultative manner, to determine the appropriate nursing care standard for each clinical unit. Productivity is measured as a percentage as follows:

Standard/actual = ____%

The budget process

Before embarking on a budget plan, it is essential to do a market survey and market projection. These are based on the organisation's strategic business plans and specific areas of growth or expansion. Strategic directions are needed by departmental managers in preparing their individual budgets. Usually the finance department or chief financial officer prepares the schedule for the budget process. This includes budget submission deadlines, review meetings, and final approval. The process can take a few months to complete. In many companies the fiscal year is from January to December. Table 17.3, page 206, illustrates an example of a budget schedule.

Once an organisation has established its goals, objectives, and specific targets for the coming fiscal year, managers can start their budget plans. Most budgets are developed for a one-year period. There are limitations on the resources available in any healthcare organisation, and budgets therefore often cannot be accepted or approved as submitted. Some needs will be more crucial than others. However, there will be opportunities for all managers to defend their proposed budgets and to engage in negotiations.

Eventually, several budget revisions will be made, and a budget will be agreed that is acceptable to top management. The budget might be far from ideal, but it represents management's attempt to accomplish its overall organisational goals for the year. The completed budget is submitted to the board of directors (or similar body) for review and approval. All budgets are reviewed in relation to the priorities and business needs of the organisation, and a nurse manager might not necessarily receive all that has been requested during the budget process. The nurse manager needs to distinguish between the needs of the organisation and the needs of departmental core services, and then make the required cuts in the planned budget.

Table 17.3 Example of budget schedule for fiscal year

Activities	From	To	Duration
1. Volume projection (marketing and revenue)	07 Aug	20 Aug	2 weeks
2. Capital budget projection and approval	07 Aug	28 Aug	3 weeks
3. Operating and personnel budget projection (by divisional and departmental managers)	05 Sep	16 Sep	2 weeks
4. Budget review meetings (1st and 2nd passes)	24 Sep	04 Oct	2 weeks
5. Finalised budgets for submission to the chief finance officer	by 06 Oct		
6. Presentation of budget to managing director	on 09 Oct		
7. Presentation of budget to executive committee	on 23 Oct		
8. Circulation of budget to board of directors	by 01 Nov		
9. Board of directors meeting to approve budget	12 Nov		

Author's creation, adapted from Parkway Group Healthcare, Singapore

The budget approval process is a dynamic function, and ongoing discussions should take place between the nurse manager and senior management to address needs and priorities.

The final step in the budget process is control and feedback. Control implies regular review of the planned budget in comparison with the actual budget. Budget control centres around variance analysis—that is, determining the underlying causes of differences between the planned budget and the actual results. Information about actual results provides feedback for future budget planning.

'The budget approval process is a dynamic function involving ongoing discussions between the nurse manager and senior management.'

Variance analysis

The difference between the actual results and planned budget is a variance—the amount by which the results vary from that which was budgeted. Variance analysis is used to evaluate the performance of units (or departments) and their managers. It is important to understand why variances occur in the current month, so that actions can be taken to prevent unfavourable or negative variances in the coming months. Variances also aid in future budget planning, so that improvements and more accurate projections can be made.

Nurse managers must investigate and understand the causes of variances. Variances can be caused by internal factors or external factors. *Internal variances* include efficiency of nurses in relation to workload—for example, some wards are able to adjust their staffing schedule when workload increases without resorting to hiring part-time staff, whereas other wards need to hire additional staff. *External variances* include changes in patient volume. Higher patient volume or workload does not necessarily result in higher revenue as it might involve higher expenses. When patient volume falls below budget, expenses are expected to decrease correspondingly. However, if this does not happen, a nurse manager must evaluate the unit's performance in terms of expense control.

'Nurse managers must investigate and understand the causes of variances.'

Variance reports are given by the finance department to nurse managers so that they can justify the variances. Finance personnel need to understand what is happening—with a view to controlling future results as much as possible. Variance analyses or reports should not be confrontational or seen as a defensive justification. Understanding why variances occur helps a manager, department, and organisation to improve its efficiency through better cost controls. However, to use budgets for control, the organisation must assign responsibility for variances to individual managers and departments.

The focus of variance analysis is on the current month, although the 'year-to-date' information should also be reviewed. A nurse manager's primary variance analysis effort is mainly directed towards expenses—because nurse managers usually have a greater degree of control over expenses than they do over revenues. An example of a variance report is shown in Table 17.4 (page 208).

'Nurse managers usually have a greater degree of control over expenses than they do over revenues.'

Table 17.4 Example of a variance report for a delivery suite

Current month	Actual	Budget	Variance	% variance	Prior month	Prior year
Deliveries	311	362	−51	−14.1%	314	347
Gross revenues	$160 416	$169 088	−$8 672	−7.7%	$139 477	$182 297
Other operating revenues	$135	$99	$36	36.4%	$15	$300
Total revenue	$160 551	$169 187	−$8 636	−5.1%	$139 492	$182 597
Salaries and benefits	$80 922	$85 836	$4 914	5.7%	$87 234	$81 196
Controllable variables	$12 551	$12 717	$166	1.3%	$12 497	$12 221
Controllable fixed	$281	$1 330	$1 049	78.9%	$462	$2 160
Non-controllable	$9 104	$9 281	$177	1.9%	$9 082	$8 676
Total expenses	$102 858	$109 164	$6 306	5.8%	$109 275	$104 255
Net operating margin	$57 693	$60 023	−$2 330	21.7%	$30 217	$78 342
% of revenue	35.9%	35.5%	0.5%	1.3%	21.7%	42.9%

Author's creation

In the example of a variance report shown in Table 17.4, the decrease in the number of deliveries corresponds with a decrease in both gross revenues and expenses. In terms of expense control, this unit's controllable variables decreased by only 1.3%, although total revenue decreased by 5.1%. The nurse manager needs to investigate which controllable expense items could be better controlled—because these expenses have increased in comparison with a year ago.

The variance report also gives the manager information on the financial performance of the unit in relation to the previous month and previous year, so that he or she can analyse the reasons for the favourable or unfavourable variances. The current month's performance in Table 17.4 appears to be better than the previous month, despite the slight decrease in deliveries; the percentage of revenue is 35.9% compared with previous month's percentage of revenue of 21.7%. Efficient management involves investigating and evaluating variances on a regular and frequent basis, and taking action to correct the variances if possible. Managerial expertise and judgment are required to evaluate and understand the variances. Flexible budget variance analysis segregates the variance into components, and allows the manager to explain why the variance occurred.

Financial management—a large part of which is variance analysis—must be considered in perspective. Quality of patient care is also critical; performance should be measured by both financial and non-financial measures. Non-financial measures include patient satisfaction, quality of care, nurse satisfaction, and innovation.

'Quality of patient care is critical; performance should be measured by both financial and non-financial measures.'

Current issues and future directions

The allocation of nursing resources is a major issue because nursing care is perceived to be expensive, and a shortage of nurses is a problem in many Western countries. A nurse manager's role in financial management can be influenced by staffing levels, effective and efficient levels of staffing, differentiated nursing practice, and the relationship of staffing to patient outcomes.

Remuneration and financial incentives for nurses represent another pressing issue. What is the impact of compensation (that is, salaries and bonuses) on productivity? The cost/benefit ratio (or cost-effectiveness) of nursing care is also an important issue. What is the cost-effectiveness of unlicensed healthcare assistants and of nursing-care delivery models?

Finally, the need to control nursing costs and cost of care continues to be a challenge for both nurse executives and nurse managers.

The role of the chief nurse executive or director of nursing is likely to expand in both strategic planning and financial management. Nursing is expected to play a key role in both the preparation of the budget and the business-planning process. Nursing-management courses are proliferating, with many programs including subjects on budgeting, financial management, and human-resource management. Nurse managers of the future will certainly need to be competent in financial management and business acumen.

As the chief nurse executive assumes a greater role in financial decision-making, nursing units will be run more like small businesses in which nurse managers will have greater empowerment and accountability for managing their budgets. This will include more authority over staffing allocations, compensation, and responsibility for revenue.

In understanding the budgeting process and its role in the planning, delivery, and evaluation of patient care, nurse managers will undoubtedly assist the hospital's bottom line by making sound financial decisions.

Conclusion

Planning, implementing, and monitoring a unit's budget requires a basic understanding of budgetary concepts (Grohar-Murray & DiCroce 2003). The nurse manager's role in financial management will vary from organisation to organisation. However, knowledge of the budget process is critical to the planning and control functions of a manager. Managers need to understand fiscal terminology, and are accountable to the organisation for maintaining a cost-effective unit. The ability to forecast unit fiscal needs with sensitivity to the organisation's economic performance is a high-level management function.

Nurse managers today are challenged to articulate their units' needs so as to ensure sufficient funds are obtained for adequate nursing staff, supplies, and equipment. Other leadership skills required in fiscal management include flexibility, creativity, and vision

'Leadership skills required in fiscal management include flexibility, creativity, and vision with regard to future needs.'

with regard to future needs. An effective leader is able to anticipate budget constraints and act proactively. Despite constraints in fiscal resources, nurse managers and leaders need to be creative in identifying alternatives to meet patient needs without compromising quality and patient safety. Nurse managers must be assertive and defend their budget requirements in a proactive and professional manner.

Chapter 18

Managing Information

Alan Scarborough

Introduction

All managers rely on information to make decisions. It is therefore essential that nurse managers understand how to use information effectively. Although it has sometimes been suggested that managers could avoid using a computer (Robbins & Mukerji 1994), times have changed and managers have become more dependent on computers. Indeed, they complain if they are denied access to up-to-date information systems. In the past, nurses have tended to see technology as dehumanising and counterproductive to the art and science of nursing. However, those now entering the nursing profession have been educated with computers, and are aware of the possibilities that the Internet and other computer information systems can provide. Attitudes have shifted within the modern nursing workforce (Richards 2001).

Information can be obtained in many forms—including personal observations, verbal interactions, written reports, and statistical information of various sorts. Information is a vital aspect of management, and modern nurse managers must be able to understand and use computer information systems.

Management functions

The French industrialist Fayol (1916) suggested that all managers perform five management functions—planning, organising, commanding, coordination, and controlling. For the nurse manager these functions can be described in the following terms.

▶ *Planning* involves the development of budgets and associated staffing plans (and the coordination of these activities).

▶ *Organising* involves the determination of what tasks are to be done, who will perform these tasks, and how reports will be provided.

▶ *Commanding* and *coordination* (taken together) involve the motivation of subordinates and the communication of decisions (often referred to as *leading*).

▶ *Controlling* involves the monitoring of performance and making the appropriate changes to meet objectives.

The last of these—controlling—is worthy of further exploration. *Controlling* can be defined as the process of monitoring activities to ensure that they are being accomplished as planned, and the correcting of any significant deviations (Robbins & Mukerji 1994). Control thus has a number of components including:

▶ setting standards and objectives;

▶ measuring performance;

▶ comparing results against these standards and objectives; and

▶ taking corrective action.

These tasks, especially the measurement of performance, lend themselves to the use of information systems. Performance is measured by collecting information of various types—including personal observations and reports of various kinds (statistical, oral, and written). Each form has particular strengths and weaknesses, but a combination of these types of information increases the probability of receiving reliable information. The use of computers has provided easier access to statistical information, and nurse managers increasingly rely on this form of information for measuring performance.

What is measured is more critical to the control process than *how* that measurement occurs, and this determines the direction of the organisation. The selection of the wrong criteria can result in serious consequences—because *what* is measured often determines what people in the organisation will attempt to excel at. This can mean that other outputs (many of them important) are neglected (Robbins & Mukerji 1994).

'*What* is measured is more critical to the control process than *how* that measurement occurs.'

Some measures are applicable to all managers. For example, because all managers direct the activities of others, criteria such as staff satisfaction, turnover, and absenteeism are often measured. In addition, most nurse managers have budgets for their areas of responsibility. Keeping costs within budget is, therefore, a fairly common control measure. Other areas of interest might include nursing costs per patient day, costs per procedure, theatre return rates, and mortality and morbidity rates.

Data versus information

Although it is commonly said that '*knowledge* is power', it is more accurate to say that '*the ability to collect and transform data into useful information* is power'. The collection and transformation of data into useful information is how knowledge is produced. To achieve this, nurse managers need to understand and use computers and information systems. One of the advantages of using computers is their ability to sort, analyse, and manipulate vast amounts of data to produce meaningful information. It is this characteristic that makes computers so useful for the nurse manager (Simpson 1997).

'The ability to collect and transform data into useful information is power.'

There is a difference between *data* and *information*. *Data* are raw unanalysed facts (such as numbers, names, or quantities). In this form, they are relatively useless to managers (Robbins & Mukerji 1994). For example, managers often collect data on the rate of absenteeism. These data do not become *information* until the data are sorted and analysed—in the form of averages, trends, and comparisons with other groups and organisations.

To be useful, information should be (Collins & McLaughlin 1996; O'Brien 1999):

▶ succinct (but accurate);
▶ complete;
▶ relevant;
▶ easily disseminated;
▶ appropriate to the needs of the recipient;
▶ understandable; and
▶ delivered on time.

Any deficiencies in one or more of these elements can render the information useless, and can lead to a poor decision being made. If information is created from inaccurate data, the information will also be inaccurate. The phrase 'garbage in; garbage out' was coined to describe this phenomenon.

A nurse manager who provides some inaccurate information to senior managers might also create suspicion about the reliability of other information. It is therefore essential that all information is checked for accuracy before passing it on or before decisions are made on the basis of such information. This can often be achieved by looking for obvious errors (for example, if the figures are significantly higher or lower than expected), or by comparing data elements with those already known.

Most health services are 'data rich but information poor'. This occurs because there is usually a huge amount of data collected by various systems, and because it is not sorted and analysed effectively.

> 'Most health services are data rich but information poor.'

Computer information systems

The term 'computer information system' refers to the production of information using the model of a 'computer within a system'. This model involves inputs, processes, and outputs. The inputs of the system are data, which are then processed through the use of various resources, including computers. The output is in the form of information. The computer itself is not the information system; rather, it is the primary piece of hardware used within the system. The software harnesses the power of the computer to turn data into information.

Nurse managers utilise information from various computer information systems, including clinical-information systems, and management-information systems.

Components

The fundamental components of a computer information system are:
- the people;
- the hardware;
- the software;
- the data; and
- the network resources.

Each of these is discussed below.

People

People are the most important components of any system. If people do not function well, the system will also be dysfunctional. It is more difficult to fix the deficiencies in people than it is to fix other components in the system. It is therefore imperative that the people who are to perform the information-management tasks are selected through a sound recruitment and selection process. The nurse manager is often involved in the selection process for these employees.

> 'People are the most important components of any system.'

The people involved are: (i) those who work within the information-system departments; and (ii) those who use the system (also called 'end-users'). Nurses and other end-users must be able to use the system, because the organisation usually relies on them to enter accurate and reliable data. Training is therefore critical to the integrity of any information system.

Hardware

Hardware can be defined as any piece of physical equipment that performs: (i) input; (ii) output; (iii) processing; and (iv) storage functions. *Input devices* are a means by which data and instructions are fed into a computer; a keyboard is the most common form of input device. *Output devices* are the means by which a computer supplies information to a user; monitors and printers are the most common forms of output device. *Processing* occurs through the central processing unit (CPU). This controls the flow of information and is where the main memory of the computer is located. A *storage device* is any device that stores information—such as the hard drive, CD-ROMs, and other disk drives.

Hardware is becoming smaller and more powerful, and it is becoming more common for nurses to view information including their rosters from a hand-held device—especially if working in a remote location.

Components of a computer information system

The fundamental components of a computer information system are:
* the people;
* the hardware;
* the software;
* the data; and
* the network resources.

Software

Software is the collective name for programs that instruct a computer to perform tasks. The main software packages used by managers include: (i) word-processing programs; (ii) spreadsheets; (iii) databases; and (iv) communication packages. *Word-processing packages* allow the manager to write, edit, and update documents more efficiently. *Spreadsheets* facilitate the analysis of large amounts of data. *Databases* organise a large amount of data and convert this into readily accessible information. *Communication packages* pass information from one computer terminal to another. The most common form of this is email, which has dramatically changed communication within and between organisations. Web browsers allow computers to interact with the Internet.

Network

A *network* connects several computers to a central system, allowing people to interact using the same data and information from different computers. A network might exist within one health facility or between the elements of an organisation that is geographically divided (even between different states or continents). In any network, the ability of different elements (perhaps using different systems) to communicate with each other is essential. System integration is therefore imperative if services are to communicate, and if data are to be freely accessed. The most common method of system integration is now via the Internet, often using wireless networks and hand-held devices (Murchison 1999).

Uses of computer information systems

Nurse managers use various types of computer information systems to extract clinical and management information to assist in decision-making. The management of information is becoming increasingly important in improving the health of individual patients and the total population for which a healthcare organisation is responsible (FitzHenry 1998). The main uses of computer information systems include:

> 'The management of information is becoming increasingly important in improving the health of individual patients and populations.'

▶ clinical management;
▶ resource management;
▶ communication; and
▶ knowledge management.
Each of these is discussed below.

Clinical management

Clinical management involves decision-making and the tracking of clinical input and outcomes—both in terms of individual patients and the wider population. This information can be categorised by diagnosis or by geography (for example, ward or service area). Clinical information systems allow the input of clinical data to be processed—thus producing clinical information.

Clinicians can use this information to monitor their activities and patient outcomes. The information is also useful for nurse managers in measuring quality outcomes and costing nursing services down to the patient level (Kaufman & Paulanka 1994). This provides nurse managers with information for developing budgets as well as indicating how much nursing costs. The ability of the system to aggregate data from the patient level to the population level is an important advantage for clinicians and managers alike (Styffe 1997).

Clinical information systems improve communication and provide greater accuracy and easier retrieval of information. Clinical information systems are also able to provide managers with a number of useful data sets that can be used for quality-improvement activities.

Uses of computer information systems

The main uses of a computer information system are:
- clinical management;
- resource management;
- communication; and
- knowledge management.

Resource management

Resource management is the allocation and monitoring of human and other resources, including goods and services. Information systems can assist nurse managers in this area by allowing the input of management data to be processed into management information. It is vital that nurse managers understand what information they require, and in what format. To ensure that the system meets their needs and the needs of the organisation, nurse managers need to be involved in the design and implementation of any management information system (FitzHenry 1998).

'Nurse managers need to be involved in the design and implementation of any management information system.'

A management information system produces information that supports many day-to-day decisions. This information includes reports and displays that managers have specified in advance (O'Brien 1999). These reports can be of three types.

▶ *Periodic reports* use a predetermined format to provide managers with information on a regular basis. A typical example is a monthly financial statement.

▶ *Exception reports* are reports that are produced only when exceptional circumstances occur—for example, if absenteeism rises to a level greater than a predefined limit. The advantage of this is that it promotes 'management by exception'—thus reducing the overwhelming amount of information otherwise required in periodic reports.

▶ *Demand reports* are the provision of information whenever the manager requests information. This provides immediate responses to questions or customised reports quickly.

Communication

Millions of people now rely on electronic mail (email) for *communication*. The first thing that many managers do when commencing work is to check their email. Full-featured email software has the ability to send messages to multiple users with predefined mailing lists, and to provide password security, automatic message forwarding, and remote user access. It also allows the storage of messages in folders as accessible records when required.

The use of email by nurse managers has increased because of its speed, reliability, convenience, and low costs (Hughes & Pakieser 1999). The disadvantages of email are the large number of messages it generates and the ease with which people can add others to their distribution lists (Feldman 2000).

Although email is a fast method of communicating, it does not communicate non-verbal messages in the same way as face-to-face communication. It should not therefore be used for the following (Davidhizar and Shearer 1999):

▶ solving complex problems;
▶ communicating when a negative relationship exists;
▶ providing an apology; and
▶ communicating negative information.

Problems with the use of email include (Tapp 2001):

▶ confidentiality,
▶ its potential for use as documentary evidence; and
▶ misuse resulting in disciplinary action.

With regard to *confidentiality*, nurse managers should always be aware that email communications are susceptible to unauthorised access by third parties.

They should be particularly aware of this issue if sending confidential or sensitive information via email. Consent should be gained from patients before healthcare information is transmitted by email. This consent should include the provision of information regarding the risks and alternative transmission methods.

'Consent should be gained from patients before healthcare information is transmitted by email.'

It is important to realise that email messages are *documents*, and that emails can be used as *evidence* in legal proceedings. This is of particular concern given that many email users believe that their messages will be seen only by the intended recipient. Messages are therefore often more candid than would normally be sent in a letter. Often the message is written hastily, is unedited, and reflects the author's true thoughts.

Many employees believe that email of a personal nature is a personal matter without any consequence—even if sent during working hours. There have been many cases in which employees have been disciplined over personal emails involving jokes and inappropriate language, and some have resulted in termination of employment. *Disciplinary* action is often supported by a policy prohibiting the use of company computer systems for personal use. If such a policy is in existence, nurse managers should ensure that all nurses with email access are aware of the policy and that they have signed the agreement. This policy should clearly state the organisation's expectations and requirements with respect to the use of email (Martinez 1997). The policy should address such issues as:

▶ not engaging in wilful and malicious activities;
▶ not sending, receiving, and accessing pornographic materials;
▶ not using abusive, profane, racist, sexist, or other objectionable language in public or private messages; and
▶ not sending messages that are unrelated to work.

These policies discourage unproductive employee behaviour (by discouraging the use of the Internet and email for activities not related to business), and they remind employees that email is employer property that can be monitored.

Problems with email

Problems with the use of email include:
- confidentiality;
- its potential for use as documentary evidence; and
- misuse resulting in disciplinary action.

Knowledge management

The collection and retrieval of information is important to *knowledge management*. Information can be stored on local computers, networks, and company Intranets. The ultimate knowledge system is the Internet. Managers can use the Internet to access large amounts of information to assist in their decision-making and to undertake formal and informal education. The key is to be able to filter the useful information from that which is unreliable.

Concerns

As discussed above, computer information systems have numerous advantages. However, there are also certain concerns. These include: (i) information overload from the sheer volume of information that is available; (ii) the potential for unauthorised access of confidential information; and (iii) costs and time.

Information overload

Managers are always looking for more information in order to make better decisions, and this can mean that information overload can become a major problem with the potential to cripple decision-making. Nurse managers are bombarded every day with requests for all sorts of information—statistics, facts, and advice regarding decisions reached—and they are expected to have this information at their fingertips. The quantity of data that has to be dealt with and disseminated simply cannot be handled manually (Simpson 1997).

'Information overload can become a major problem with the potential to cripple decision-making.'

The 'more-is-better myth' was explored by Robbins & Mukerji (1994). This myth has two components. The first is that a greater quantity of information will necessarily lead to better decisions. The second is that managers need all the information they request. Neither statement is true. An increased quantity of information might not lead to better decisions because:

▶ a manager can become overwhelmed with information;
▶ the value of any information depends on more than mere quantity; and
▶ a manager who has the relevant data might not understand how it fits together.

The nurse manager therefore needs to be selective in what information is requested and what information is used in decision-making.

Privacy, confidentiality, and security

Although the terms 'privacy', 'confidentiality', and 'security' are often used interchangeably, they are separate entities. *Privacy* refers primarily to the right of individuals to determine when, how, and to what extent information is transmitted. *Confidentiality* is trust that the information that has been shared will be respected and used only for the purpose disclosed. *Security* is the protection of information from accidental or intentional access by unauthorised people—including modification or destruction of the information (Mulligan 1998).

Modern methods of electronic data storage and distribution of patient information present new challenges in the task of protecting confidentiality. At the same time, demands for 'seamless' care that crosses organisational boundaries, and an awareness of the treatment errors that can result from a failure to transfer information effectively, have generated incentives to create new electronic linkages and to reduce barriers in the transfer of patient data. Protecting the patient medical record in the information age is therefore difficult. Computerisation has profound implications for privacy, security and confidentiality, and these implications must be proactively explored and acted upon

'Computerisation has profound implications for privacy, security and confidentiality,'

through the development of effective preventative measures (Styffe 1997).

Costs and time

The cost of computer information systems is an ongoing issue. The hardware has only a short life, and information systems require more and more resources to turn data into information. The collection of information is always at some cost in terms of hardware and software utilised, and in terms of the time people take to collect and analyse the data. A cost/benefit analysis should always be made when requesting any type of information.

Concerns with computer information systems

The main concerns with the use of computer information systems are:
- information overload;
- privacy, confidentiality, and security; and
- costs and time.

Conclusion

All managers rely on information to make decisions, and nurse managers must understand how to use information effectively. The vast (and growing) amount of information that is available, and the daily requirement to manage this information effectively and efficiently, mean that the modern nurse manager must be able to understand and use computer information systems with confidence.

Chapter 19

The Nurse Manager as Educator

Sue Frost

Introduction

There is a global shortage of qualified nurses, and health services are recruiting nurses from across the world. Nurses are 'knowledge workers' who have a primary loyalty to the profession. With respect to this concept of 'knowledge workers', Stewart (2003, p. 101) has observed:

> At the same time that employers have weakened the ties of job security and loyalty, they more than ever depend on human capital . . . they [knowledge workers] bring to their work not only their bodies but their minds—even their souls—and are far more loyal to their work.

Nurses, as 'knowledge workers', will stay committed to their employers if they are provided with the resources for interesting work, and if they are able to learn, grow, and use all of their skills. If such an environment is not forthcoming, nurses, like other knowledge workers, will move on. This presents nurse managers with challenges in creating environments in which nurse practitioners can flourish and perform effectively.

'In the process of learning, skills and competence complement knowledge and understanding.'

Nurse managers must therefore facilitate *learning* among their staff. In the process of learning, skills and competence complement knowledge and understanding to improve performance and effective practice.

Many nurses believe that learning is simply about 'knowing the right thing to do'. Learning is seen as an *outcome*, whereby the practitioner gains understanding that serves as a foundation for professional 'knowing'. However, Komives and Woodard (1996, p. 219) argued that learning is also a *process* that:

> . . . focuses on the kind of strategies people use to solve new problems, how they respond to feedback and information, how they gather and interpret data, how they determine its relevance and how strong the evidence needs to be before they are satisfied they can make a decision or solve a problem.

One of the defining characteristics of professional practice is *active* learning— a continuum of developing knowledge and understanding, and of building skill through solving problems.

Deep and surface learning

People can be said to learn in three ways (Entwhistle 1996):

▶ surface learning;
▶ strategic learning; and
▶ deep learning.

Surface learners focus on facts as if they were self-explanatory rules to be followed. *Strategic learners* learn whatever is needed 'to get by today'. In contrast to these first two types of learners, *deep learners* try to make connections between new ideas and their previous learning. Such deep learners construct meaning in ways that are capable of continuous development and capable of being transferred to different applications. Practitioners who are deep learners think laterally, find a range of solutions, know how to make choices, and reject inappropriate practice.

Although nurses do need to be up to date with latest techniques, they need to know more than current procedures and protocols. Rather, they need to be part of a *learning organisation*. Learning organisations encourage nurses to learn from their own experience. Such organisations provide nurses with opportunities to: (i) review, critique, and question their day-to-day practice; (ii) try new ideas

while drawing on the literature and
the experience of others; and (iii)
take ownership of their contribution
to the care program. All of this
requires the skills of deep learning,

'Nurses need to be part of a
learning organisation.'

logical thinking, and critical reasoning. It also requires space and time to
question, reflect, and discuss.

Single-loop and double-loop learning

According to Argyris (1991), 'most people define learning too narrowly as mere
"problem solving", so they focus on identifying and correcting errors in the
external environment'. This 'single-loop' learning does not support a sustained
knowledge base. Such learning comes from 'double-loop' (reflective) learning.
As Argyris (2000) put it:

> Solving problems is important. But if learning is to persist, [learners] need
> to reflect critically on their own behaviour, identify the ways they often
> inadvertently contribute to the organisation's problems and then change
> how they act.

Managers have a key role in supporting nurses to learn from experience. The
role of the manager as educator is not simply to make appropriate courses of study
available. Helping nurses to learn reflectively is more likely to create a workforce
that responds to change, anticipates issues, and creates a dynamic approach with
patients at the heart of care. Wedderburn Tate (1999) challenged the nurse
manager in the following terms: 'When you examine your behaviour as a leader,
what do you see?'. Wedderburn Tate (1999) also asked the following questions
of the manager:

▶ Do you consciously or unconsciously court 'single-loop' or 'double-loop'
  learning?
▶ Do you hold on to a belief or idea even when the 'sell-by' date is past?
▶ Do you accept that your plans are always subject to change?
▶ How do you respond to criticism?
▶ What life position do you adopt?

In contemporary health care, nurses must apply their knowledge and skills
in complex and changing environments. They deal with problems that do not
have simple solutions, are increasingly required to supervise others in the
delivery of complex regimens of care, and are often responsible for several such
regimens simultaneously. The manager has an important role in providing a

LIVERPOOL JOHN MOORES UNIVERSITY
LEARNING & INFORMATION SERVICES

learning environment that supports skill development in the care of a number of patients with complex and challenging problems.

Creating learning opportunities

Levi Strauss, one of the most successful businesses in the world, spends four out of every five dollars on 'knowing', rather than on 'doing'. However, when the United Kingdom Nursing and Midwifery Council introduced a mandatory requirement for nurses to spend five days in every three years on professional updating (NMC 1993), there was concern about whether this could be afforded! It can be difficult to allocate resources to the maintenance of up-to-date practice. However, nurse managers need to think about the way in which education provides a coherent framework for the development of the individual in terms of knowledge and understanding—rather than seeing education simply as a funding issue (see Figure 19.1, below).

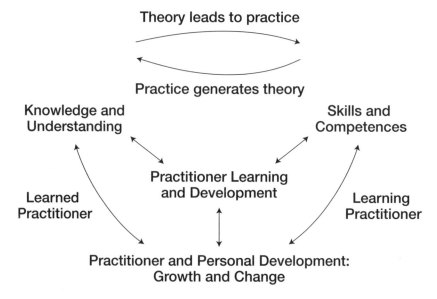

Figure 19.1 A framework of practitioner learning
Richard Graham, University of Huddersfield; published with permission

Theory and practice are inseparable. When nurses are practising they are using, testing, and building theory. And when they are learning theory, they are examining it for its applicability to practice. In developing learning opportunities, nurse managers must recognise and enhance this relationship between theory and practice.

The English National Board for Nursing, Midwifery and Health Visiting (ENB 1995) has identified the characteristics of successful nursing environments as follows:

- managers who champion learning;
- work programs that enable all staff members to maintain their development;
- challenging and questioning practitioners;
- reflective practice embedded in clinical supervision;
- learning activities (including journal clubs, seminars, and review meetings);
- personal development plans in place;
- planned investment in staff learning as part of the organisational plan; and
- nurse leaders with a commitment to their own development.

Learning logs and portfolios

Students often spend time scribbling notes during formal lectures, seminars, or handovers. The challenge is to encourage students to use *learning logs* as a way of managing their learning. A learning log involves noting down things that are puzzling or interesting, or taking note of things to do. A learning log is a way of organising the things to be thought about, checked, and pursued.

One way of encouraging practitioners to use a learning log is to try it out during a handover report in a clinical setting. Nurse managers and their staff members can take note of things that should be thought about later, checked on, or followed up in some other way. This is done in a book separate from the regular information that informs the daily work routine. These notes and reflections can contribute to the reflective element of a personal portfolio used in a review of professional and personal development needs.

Learning sets—how to learn from one another

Another device to support learning is the use of action learning sets. These are formal learning groups in which each participant contributes in ways that enable colleagues to learn from one another. The learning agenda is agreed upon by the group, and each member of the learning set has time allocated that can be used in a variety of ways—depending on the issues and challenges that he or she wishes to bring to the learning set. Learning sets can be used to achieve the following:

❯ making progress towards the solution of a real problem;

❯ determining how to approach an ill-defined problem to which nobody knows the answer (or even an appropriate course of action); and

❯ creating an environment in which practitioners learn with, and from, each other in the pursuit of their common tasks.

Learning sets often operate best when immediate colleagues are not in the same group. The manager can help to establish sets in which colleagues from different settings can learn from one another. Indeed, a core principle is that the manager should also participate in learning that challenges and reflects his or her own practice.

> 'The nurse manager should participate in learning that challenges and reflects his or her own practice.'

Using skills escalators—the skills inventory

The concept of a 'skills escalator' underpins some national strategies to develop the health workforce. The concept is usually linked with notions of lifelong learning whereby staff members are encouraged to participate in renewing and extending their skills. A policy to establish skills escalator programs in healthcare services is underpinned by the notion that: '. . . all staff are encouraged through a strategy of lifelong learning to constantly renew and extend their skills and knowledge, enabling them to move up the escalator' (DoH 2003). The core principle is that clinical staff in all disciplines and at all levels should be supported with a framework that focuses on the necessary skills to do the job required. This might include 'customer care' skills for an admissions nurse or doctor, or computer skills for clinicians working in services with electronic patient records.

Managers are responsible for providing the framework in which such skills development can operate. This can commence with the provision of on-the-job vocational training, progress to formal professional programs, and extend to continuing professional development. The notion is that learners can step on or off the skills escalator at any time, and receive recognition for the level that they have achieved.

A skills inventory is a technique for establishing an agreement (among a manager, a practitioner, and an educator) on the skills that are central to the role of the practitioner. The intention is that all parties then support the development of skills in the practice environment of the practitioner.

This enables the skills escalator to be accessed appropriately as part of a longer-term plan.

Formal programs—what courses offer

Formal courses and programs are the most common approach to the development of staff learning. Formal courses of study offer an opportunity to learn with others—often supported by a significant library and other resources of learning materials. Such learning is often assessed and accredited.

It is essential that nurse managers be clear about the outcomes that are expected from a given course of study, and that measurable results are available to assess the investment made in staff.

Table 19.1 Assessment of courses

Aims and characteristics of course	Is this the right course for my staff?
Improve knowledge	What new things will staff members learn?
Improve skills	What new things will staff members be able to do as a result of this course?
Improve confidence and responsibility	How will personal behaviour change?
Location	Where does study take place? Is this education at the point of need?
Resources of course	What resources and facilities will be available to my staff?
Timescale of course	How long will the course take to complete?
Level of course	Does this build on existing skills?
Credentialling for course	What qualification or professional recognition will the course give? How will this add to the credentialling of the workforce?
Skill mix covered by course	How will the course contribute to the nursing skill mix in our setting?
Strategic and operational aspects of course	Does this course enable the service to meet its goals, care for new patients, and offer better services to patients?

Author's creation

A nurse manager must ensure that the program is likely to meet the needs of the organisation and the individual, both professionally and intellectually. It is useful to identify the results that might be expected from what is often a high-cost investment. Table 19.1 (page 229) provides a checklist of questions that can be asked in assessing the merits of any proposed course.

Mentoring and coaching

Mentoring and coaching relationships are not only useful in achieving work goals, but also provide an important support for practitioner development. This is part of the general concept of clinical supervision, but with a definite emphasis on staff development.

Nurse managers have a responsibility to help staff members find an appropriate mentor or coach. One approach is to be explicit with staff members about how the nurse manager makes personal use of a mentor.

A nurse manager can often act as a coach—with a focus on how the individual can contribute to the team's performance. However, mentorship is more likely to focus on individual needs. The mentoring process involves coaching, advising, career guidance, and counselling. As Owen (2001, p. 126) has observed: 'The mentor cares about the individual and acts as a guide'.

Role modelling

As an educator, the nurse manager is a role model. If the manager is committed to his or her own personal development and education, colleagues are more likely to be enthused about education.

Many people gain a great deal from the experiences and stories of others, particularly their manager. Nurses transmit a lot of their knowledge and skill through the stories they tell. The manager can, in effect, become a powerful 'co-author' in helping staff members to shape their practice through learning from one another's stories. One approach is to invite senior nurses from outside to come to talk to staff in the form of a 'master class'. These are powerful mediators of culture, role expectations, and performance.

On-the-job training and teaching in clinical settings

Nurse managers and educators frequently talk about the importance of practice-based learning, but they often fail to exploit the real opportunities that it provides. This is partly because most clinical settings are focused on 'getting the work done'. The systematic planning of care can become yet another task in itself—thus losing the value of systematic planning as a vehicle for team decision-making.

The challenges that must be overcome in developing effective learning in the clinical setting are:

▶ using theory to explain practice;
▶ allowing space and time for teaching;
▶ involving the patient in the teaching session in a meaningful way;
▶ taking risks; and
▶ enabling nurses to learn from all members of the team (including unqualified staff and those from other disciplines).

Reducing the clinical–academic divide

For many years, nurses have argued over ways by which the perceived divide between theory and practice can be reduced. There remains an inaccurate perception that education is dislocated from practice. Part of the problem relates to the routine and rhythm of two worlds that use different languages, have different priorities, and even have different functional years.

Unlike other professions, nursing continues to criticise its intellectual status and to relegate its education to being 'out of touch' with the real world. There are several ways in which this divide can be reduced. These essentially involve working partnerships between healthcare providers and healthcare educators. Effective approaches to reducing the theory–practice divide include the following:

▶ supporting students in practice-based learning;
▶ whole-systems planning for education and practice; and
▶ joint appointments and new careers.

Each of these is discussed below.

Supporting students in practice-based learning

The curriculum leading to professional qualification should respect and reflect contemporary developments in practice. Students must be fit to practise at the time of qualification, and fit for a specific purpose in a specific setting fairly quickly after qualification. Professional education must therefore reflect contemporary practice, and clinical managers have a part to play in enabling students to make connections between theory and practice when they are caring for patients in real settings.

Some managers exploit technology to support learning in the clinical workplace. Initiatives include on-line discussion with nurses in other centres, rapid access to nursing literature, on-line learning support at the nursing station, and the use of workforce-demand assessment tools in the clinical setting.

Academics and managers need to establish effective partnerships to: (i) identify what is needed from practice learning; and (ii) establish an inventory of key skills to be acquired. In this way, the limited experience available can be maximised, and students can be properly prepared to work in real settings with patients and clients.

Whole-systems planning for education and practice

The managerial concept of 'whole-systems theory' has recently been applied to the provision of education.

Applying this theory to education involves bringing together all of the stakeholders in education—including patients, nurses, managers, funders, teachers, students, and agencies. All of the processes, connections, and people involved in education are then 'mapped'. This includes policy drivers, new protocols, individual needs, and professional frameworks. The connections, gaps, nodal points, and key players are thus identified. Task groups can work on key areas of discontinuity, and problem areas can be readily identified.

'The most important aspect is a sense of joint ownership of educational development.'

Perhaps the most important aspect of such a facilitated process is the sense of joint ownership of educational development that emerges.

Joint appointments and new careers

Joint appointments have a role in uniting theory and practice. Some joint appointments have been highly successful in this respect—although the challenge of meeting competing demands is sometimes too difficult, and the dual role can become unsustainable.

The developing role of the nurse manager has education and practice as core and embedded sub-roles. Some of the most effective joint appointments in nurse management occur at a senior level where the nurse manager can influence systems that effect joint working—rather than working at an individual level within the organisation. In these senior management roles, the nurse leads, directs, and establishes a framework for clinical practice. Central to these newer roles is a responsibility to embed education and enquiry within the clinical environment.

Joint working also means that educators need to be part of the practice environment. Guidelines developed in the United Kingdom have recommended the establishment of clinical deans to support clinical academic careers by forging new partnerships between service institutions and educational institutions (CDH 1999). Other mechanisms include the development of 'clinical sabbatical' programs in which academic staff return to practice for significant periods of renewal of practice skill. In addition, agreements can be established by which clinical practitioners contribute to formal on-campus programs in return for full campus rights. Such agreements enable practitioners to gain access to mentorship and support for their clinical and educational role in the workplace.

Conclusion

Education is everybody's business, and the nurse manager has an important role to play as an educator, facilitator, and developer. If nurses are to practise effectively, the manager's role is crucial in building a learning environment.

> 'Education is everybody's business . . . the nurse manager's role is crucial in building a learning environment.'

Managing people means managing intellectual capital. Ensuring that learning becomes part of the 'day job' is a management function that can make a measurable and real difference to the patient's experience of health care. The Richards report (1977) suggested that:

> . . . responsibility within clinical governance places an obligation on service providers . . . [the] proper management and provision of initial and continuing education will be part of this obligation such that patient safety is assured, standards are maintained and accountability for teaching and learning is identified.

The educator role of nurse managers is not optional; it is a core part of the leadership role that ensures effective nursing.

Moss Kanter (1990) discussed the key elements of a strategy for organisational development. She suggested that education must follow 'five Fs':

▶ focused;
▶ fit for purpose;

▶ flexible;

▶ financially sound; and

▶ fun.

If practitioners do not enjoy learning they will not see it as a natural part of their daily routines and working lives. The nurse manager, as an educator, must ensure that learning becomes, simply, a part of the routine work.

Chapter 20

Coping with Hostility

Michael Cully

Introduction

Hostility and overt aggression have been identified as factors that have a significant influence on the delivery of clinical care (Gournay 2001) and on the recruitment and retention of staff (Jackson, Clare & Mannix 2002). Such hostility is not restricted to interactions with patients and their families; it also occurs in interactions with other staff members.

In the past, healthcare professionals have accepted aggression as being 'part of the territory' (Daldt 1981), but this is now recognised as toxic, and is actively discouraged by organisations through the promulgation of 'zero tolerance' programs (Whittingdon 2002). It is important that nurse managers be aware of these developments and that they support systems that cope adequately with the threat of hostility.

> 'It is important that nurse managers support systems that cope adequately with the threat of hostility.'

To put in place a system that protects both patients and staff, nurse managers require a sound understanding of the ways in which hostility and aggression evolve and how they can be dealt with. Nurse managers should be familiar with the policies and protocols of the facility in which they work, and should also play a major part in the ongoing development of those policies and protocols.

Predictors of hostility and aggressive behaviour

Although it is impossible to predict aggression with any certainty, there are certain populations that are more likely to be aggressive than others (RCPsych 1996), and if a person is in more than one of the 'risk' populations, the risk is cumulative. For example, if a person is identified as someone with a history of violence, is a current substance abuser, is dissatisfied with the healthcare service, and is in pain, that person is more likely to be aggressive than a person who is suffering from pain, but does not belong to the other groups.

Populations of interest include:

▶ those with a past history of aggression, particularly if the aggression has occurred in healthcare settings;
▶ those who are in pain;
▶ young, single males;
▶ those with a history of drug or alcohol abuse;
▶ elderly patients with dementia or delirium;
▶ those with organic brain pathology—hypoxia (acute or chronic) and brain trauma (cerebrovascular accident, concussion);
▶ those who are experiencing an exacerbation of mental illness;
▶ those with a learning disability; and
▶ those with a history of violence towards themselves or others.
Each of these is discussed below.

Past history of aggression

Patients with a past history of aggression, particularly if the aggression has occurred in healthcare settings, are more likely to be aggressive again. The likelihood of aggression is gauged by considering factors such as the *time* of the previous hostility (more likely if previous episode was within the past six months), the *setting* of that behaviour (more likely

'Patients with a past history of aggression, particularly if the aggression has occurred in healthcare settings, are more likely to be aggressive again.'

if previous episode occurred in a healthcare facility as opposed to a community setting), and the *type* of aggression (more likely if previous episode was physical causing injury, than if physical without injury or verbal) (CSAHS 2001).

Often the healthcare facility is the single point of reference for people seeking help. This can lead to dissatisfaction with the service, and to anger based on past experiences.

Although it is unusual, staff members also display these behaviours on occasions.

Those who are in pain

People who are in pain are more likely to be intolerant of external events that add to their distress. Events that might otherwise be considered trivial can be the stimulus for hostility or aggression.

Young single males

Young, single males are more likely to be aggressive than other populations. However, it should be noted that, in mental-health settings, women are only slightly less likely to be physically aggressive than males.

Predictors of hostility and aggressive behaviour

Certain groups of people are more likely to exhibit hostile or aggresive behaviour. Populations of interest include:

- those with a past history of aggression, particularly if the aggression has occurred in healthcare settings;
- those who are in pain;
- young, single males;
- those with a history of drug or alcohol abuse;
- elderly patients with dementia or delirium;
- those with organic brain pathology—hypoxia (acute or chronic) and brain trauma (cerebrovascular accident, concussion);
- those who are experiencing an exacerbation of mental illness;
- those with a learning disability; and
- those with a history of violence towards themselves or others.

Each of these is explored in greater detail in the text of this chapter.

Those with a history of drug or alcohol abuse

In people with a history of drug or alcohol abuse, hostility and aggression can be due to poor judgment, disorientation, or disinhibition. Alcohol intoxication is the most likely condition to be encountered, and intoxicated people are twelve times more likely to be aggressive than sober people (NSWHD 2001). Heroin addicts who are withdrawing from the drug are up to sixteen times more likely to be aggressive than other patients (NSWHD 2001).

The nurse manager should also be aware of patients who have been taking amphetamines or cocaine; both of these drugs can lead to persistent paranoid psychosis. Patients who have taken hallucinogens (such as LSD, 'ecstasy', and 'magic mushrooms') can experience anxiety and fear. There is also mounting evidence to suggest that marijuana can cause paranoia and anxiety in users (CDHA 2002).

Again it should be noted that nurses and other staff members might also take alcohol and other drugs. Indeed, they might have ingested alcohol or drugs before coming on duty.

Elderly patients with dementia or delirium

Elderly patients with dementia or delirium can have an increased tendency to hostility and aggression—especially in situations in which there is an inability to cope with the demands of hospitalisation. This can even lead to rage reactions.

It is worth noting that many elderly people passing through emergency departments are likely to be suffering from delirium caused by a systemic infection or by poisoning by prescription drugs or over-the-counter drugs. Nurses should also be aware of the fact that many cases of delirium that develop during hospitalisation go undiagnosed or are misdiagnosed (Smeltzer & Bare 2000).

Those with organic brain pathology

Patients with hypoxia (acute or chronic) or brain trauma (cerebrovascular accident, concussion, and so on) are more likely to exhibit hostile or aggressive behaviour. Any form of organic brain pathology can alter cognitive and emotional function—thus causing uncharacteristic or inappropriate behaviour.

Those who are experiencing an exacerbation of mental illness

People who are experiencing an exacerbation of mental illness can exhibit inappropriate affect, although it must be pointed out that people with a diagnosis of schizophrenia are *less likely* to be aggressive than other people. People who are suffering from auditory and visual hallucinations, delusions, and disinhibition have the potential to become aggressive. The risk of aggression is increased if hallucinations are of a 'command' nature—that is, if their content is about causing harm to others. However, if the content of hallucinations is more benign, there is no increased risk of aggression (Appelbaum, Robbins & Monahan 2000).

Although people with a diagnosed mental illness are not necessarily in a 'risk category', those who do not follow their treatment plans are.

> 'The risk of aggression is increased if hallucinations are of a 'command' nature about causing harm to others.'

Those with a learning disability

In those with a learning disability, the mechanisms underlying aggression are usually frustration or attention-seeking (Volkmar 2001). Significant mental illness is twice as likely to appear in this population (Tonge 1998). The nature of these dual conditions is poorly understood, and frequently leads to poor treatment. It is likely that some of the behaviours ascribed to learning disability should be explained in terms of untreated mental illness.

> 'It is likely that some of the behaviours ascribed to learning disability should be explained in terms of untreated mental illness.'

Among people with more severe learning disabilities, there are also obvious communication and adjustment problems associated with episodes of health care that can contribute to aggressive responses.

Those with a history of violence towards themselves or others

Patients or relatives with a history of violence towards themselves or others should always be regarded as having a high potential for violent behaviour towards others. Suicidal patients have decided to die and are prepared to kill. This combination makes them potentially dangerous to others.

Recognising imminent aggression

Outbursts of hostility or aggression are usually preceded by warning signs. By being alert to these signs, nurse managers and healthcare teams might be able to intervene at an early stage and terminate an episode before it becomes critical. Warning signs are listed in the Box on page 240.

Warning signs of imminent aggression

Warning signs of imminent aggression include the following:
- increased restlessness, bodily tension, pacing, and arousal;
- increased volume, speed, and pitch of speech; erratic or impulsive movements;
- tense and angry facial expression; signs of discontentment;
- fixed staring;
- incongruous behaviour;
- refusal to communicate, withdrawal; refusal to follow direction;
- unclear thought processes and poor concentration; (misunderstanding of situations by such people is common, with an accompanying risk of aggression that is meant to protect the confused person from the perceived threatening behaviours of carers);
- delusions or hallucinations with violent content (particularly command hallucinations directing the person to harm self or others);
- verbal threats or gestures (including invasion of personal space);
- self-reporting of angry or violent feelings by service users.

Adapted from RCPsych (2001)

Many of the behaviours listed in the Box can also be displayed by staff members, especially if they have been treated unfairly. Of course, whether the perception of unfairness is shared by the nurse manager is not relevant to this perception; the nurse might feel wronged and slighted whatever the perception of the manager might be.

The aggression cycle

An 'aggression cycle' has been described (Bowie 1989). This has implications for the management of aggression—because there are distinct strategies that can be applied to each stage of the cycle. There are five stages to the aggression cycle (Bowie 1989):
- triggering incidents;
- escalation (verbal stage);
- crisis (physical aggression);
- settling phase; and
- post-crisis depression.

Each of these is described below. However, it should be noted that this is a theoretical framework that does not always reflect reality. It is not always possible to identify a trigger, and the aggressive person might not necessarily move sequentially through all stages of the cycle. A person might not complete the cycle, might apparently jump a stage, or might revert to an earlier stage in the cycle.

The aggression cycle

The framework of this section of this chapter is based on the 'aggression cycle' (Bowie 1989).

There are five stages to the aggression cycle:
- triggering incidents;
- escalation (verbal stage);
- crisis (physical aggression);
- settling phase; and
- post-crisis depression.

This section of the chapter deals with each of these stages in turn.

1. Triggering incidents

Triggers include:
- provocation;
- response to failure;
- miscommunication;
- frustrating situations;
- violation of personal space, and
- disappointment of expectations.

Provocation

Provocations include verbal insults, insulting physical gestures, and jostling or pushing. Many assaultive patients claim that they were provoked by staff—for example, if they have had things taken from them (such as cigarettes, drink, and food).

Staff members can become hostile if they feel ignored and undervalued by frequent roster changes, if they perceive that other staff members are getting away with less work, or if they encounter a lack of respect from medical practitioners. Ineffective limit-setting and enforcement can also be provocative. These complaints indicate a need for consistency of approach—both by managers to their staff and by staff to patients and relatives.

Aggression by patients or other members of the public is often triggered by staff behaviours that are aggressive in themselves. These include:
- being inflexible and refusing to negotiate;
- using disparaging terms about others;

 ▶ assuming bad faith on the part of patients;
 ▶ lacking patience, being critical in an unconstructive way; and
 ▶ demanding, rather than requesting.

Staff members can be assaulted as a consequence of rudeness by staff members on the preceding shift. Nurse managers should ensure that staff members are educated in the principles of customer service, and that courteous and efficient service becomes the norm. It is also reasonable to suggest that staff members discuss and develop acceptable mechanisms for venting anger, frustration, anxiety, and other potentially destructive emotions that are generated by the nature of their work.

'Nurse managers should ensure that courteous and efficient service becomes the norm.'

Triggers

This section of the chapter discusses triggers to an aggressive situation. The text discusses the following triggers:

• provocation;
• response to failure;
• miscommunication;
• frustrating situations;
• violation of personal space, and
• disappointment of expectations.

Adapted from Jones (1990)

Response to failure

Response to failure is frequently a source of hostility and aggression in people who (for whatever reason) are unable to complete a task. This is common in people suffering from a cognitive deficit—in whom a combination of frustration and panic can lead to rage.

Miscommunication

Miscommunication is a common trigger for aggression, and such miscommunication is more likely to occur during routine interactions between staff and patients than in complex situations in which nurses are paying close attention to their patients.

The nurse manager should therefore ensure that simple checks of understanding are incorporated into all professional exchanges between staff and patients. These checks can be carried out by using paraphrasing and summarising techniques. For example, patients should be encouraged to paraphrase staff communication. The time taken to clarify communication is time well spent.

Frustrating situations

Frustrating situations give rise to aggression. Quality audits should always include consideration of the user-friendliness of routines and requirements. Consideration should also be given to lack of clarity in communications as being a source of frustration.

Violation of personal space

Violation of personal space is a well-recognised trigger for aggression. In Western societies, the comfortable conversational distance between people is about a metre, but concepts of personal space differ among various cultures.

As a person becomes more agitated, his or her requirements for personal space increase many times (perhaps as much as fourfold). Staff members must give an angry person more space. They also need to be aware that if they are aroused by the person's anger and/or aggression, their own need for greater personal space will grow. This can affect their ability to remain clear-headed and in control.

'Staff members must give an angry person more space.'

Disappointment of expectations

Disappointment of expectations is sometimes a euphemism for lying and/or breaking promises. It is unprofessional and unhelpful to be untruthful, or to make promises that are beyond one's capacity to keep.

In terms of negotiation, staff members must ensure that they are acting with the full knowledge and support of other staff members. Unless negotiated terms are accepted and enacted by all staff members, including the nurse manager, the patient is likely to become anxious or angry as a result of a lack of consistency.

2. Escalation stage

In the escalation phase, the aggressor is in a state of high physical and emotional arousal that equates with a 'flight-or-fight' state. Physiological functions are altered by an outpouring of adrenaline. Anger increases.

The primary aim of staff members should be to reduce the anxiety and anger by calming the person. The following strategies for calming agitated people have been identified (Turnbull & Paterson 1999):

◗ personalising;
◗ reflecting, feeling, and reassuring;
◗ using open questions;
◗ using the 'Rule of Five' to simplify and clarify communications;
◗ setting limits and negotiating;
◗ using planned ignoring of some behaviours;
◗ using personal space constructively; and
◗ offering medication.

Each of these is discussed below.

Personalising

'Depersonalising' (such as the use of personally offensive words) is often an indication of impending physical attack. It is as though the attacker is minimising the importance of his or her actions by making the victim something less than human. It is therefore important for healthcare workers to reinforce, by word and action, their own humanity and caring role. It is also important to create a larger physical space between the parties—that is, step back.

> 'Depersonalising . . . as though the attacker is minimising the importance of his or her actions by making the victim something less than human.'

Reflecting, feeling, and reassuring

Nurses should identify the feelings of the angry person and comment on them in a reassuring manner: 'I appreciate that you're angry' or 'It's understandable that you're angry'. These techniques must be tied to limit-setting (see below, page 246).

Using open questions

Open questions allow the angry person to have much greater positive input into the encounter—thus reducing the likelihood of miscommunication. Closed questions are very useful for obtaining facts, but they leave control of communication in the hands of the questioner—because the person must rely on the 'right' question being asked.

De-escalation strategies

This section of the chapter discusses strategies for the nurse manager to consider in handling aggressive situations during the escalation stage.

The text discusses the following strategies:

- personalising;
- reflecting, feeling, and reassuring;
- using open questions;
- using the 'Rule of Five' to simplify and clarify communications;
- setting limits and negotiating;
- using planned ignoring of some behaviours;
- using personal space constructively; and
- offering medication.

Adapted from Turnbull & Paterson (1999)

Using the 'Rule of Five'

The 'Rule of Five' refers to using no more than five words per sentence, and no more than five letters per word. Although it is impossible to adhere to this rule strictly, the rule is a useful reminder to keep communication simple with angry and confused people. Language should be free of jargon, free of slang, contain few qualifiers, and feature few pronouns.

Although it is relatively easy to control the use of jargon when talking to an angry person, nurses should be alert to any tendency to revert to its use when a colleague arrives on the scene. If this occurs, the angry person is effectively cut out of the communication loop.

Planned ignoring

Planned ignoring is essentially a behaviour-modification strategy in which inappropriate behaviours—such as low-level aggression—are ignored (and therefore not rewarded). The patient then provides more appropriate responses that have previously been taught to him or her by the healthcare team. To be used effectively, planned ignoring must be part of a pre-existing and agreed-upon plan of care. The patient must be:

- motivated;
- able to learn to recognise inappropriate behaviours; and
- willing to select and implement agreed-upon strategies for seeking attention.

If the patient is not included in the program, planned ignoring is not planned at all—it is *ad hoc* ignoring, and likely to escalate the situation further.

Using limits

Many healthcare facilities have policies that cover unacceptable behaviour by patients. People should be made aware of what staff members will do if unacceptable behaviours do not stop. Nurses might have to impose limits and give directions by using firm words. For example, it might be appropriate to state: 'Stop shouting; then I will listen to you'.

Negotiation

Nurses should try to negotiate mutually acceptable outcomes. It is always a good idea to have a best-possible outcome and a worst-acceptable outcome in mind. Negotiations should be limited to this range. Note that there must be unanimity of approach by healthcare staff to negotiations. All staff members must be aware of, and committed to, negotiating within the set limits.

Using space constructively

Nurses should not directly confront agitated patients. Rather, they should maintain a safe distance. It is best to stand slightly to one side—preferably the non-dominant side (which is usually the side on which a person wears a wristwatch). This assists in providing the patient with a clear escape route, and might avoid a violent confrontation.

Offering medication if prescribed

This can be a useful early intervention—particularly when dealing with cognitively impaired people whose ability to relate appropriately and predictably with others cannot be assumed. If the person is cognitively accessible, offering *oral* medication is almost always the preferred option (Allen et al. 2001).

If above strategies fail

In some instances, discretion should take precedence over valour and the nurse should withdraw. This is particularly appropriate if:

- the nurse is alone;
- the angry person refuses to leave when asked to do so;
- the nurse feels that there is no chance of regaining control; or
- the nurse feels that he or she is worsening the situation by staying.

While retreating to a safer area it is wise to remove objects that have obvious potential to be used as weapons. Nurse managers should maintain a tidy desk because pens and other tools can make potentially dangerous weapons.

Help should be summoned if the nurse manager feels that the situation is out of control. If possible, this should be done discreetly to avoid inciting violence.

Prior arrangements for emergency situations should always be in place.

Staff members must be oriented to their working environment. They must know their escape routes (and which way doors open), be aware of

'Prior arrangements for emergency situations should always be in place.'

the location of safe havens, and know how to summon help immediately (by use of duress alarms, telephones, or shouting for help). Personal alarms might be necessary—depending upon the setting. However, personal alarms should never be worn around the neck. Rather, they should be attached to a belt.

3. Crisis point

At the crisis point, negotiation and de-escalation have failed, and the angry person has become physically violent. The dominant emotion displayed by the person is hostility, and the major aim of staff members is to protect themselves and other patients. Possible strat-egies are escape, using breakaway techniques, physical or chemical restraint of the angry person, or seclusion of the person.

'Staff and other patients should be removed to areas of greater safety until control of the situation is regained.'

There is a clear need for addi-tional resources from elsewhere in the facility. Assistance from the

police service might be required (essential if the client is armed). If possible, staff and other patients should be removed to areas of greater safety until control of the situation is regained.

4. Settling phase

In this phase, the aggressor has expended his or her physical energy, and the crisis point appears to have passed. However, the person is still likely to be angry and anxious, and has the potential to return to earlier phases of the cycle.

Complex problem-solving is not an option now. Staff actions must focus on maintaining the safety of patients and staff by tending to any injuries as a first priority, keeping the aggressor in a quiet, supervised location, relieving staff as required, and using medication if necessary. If physical restraint has been applied as an intervention, it should be removed as soon as possible. A decision to remove restraint is based on the aggressor's level of cooperation and compliance.

Staff members need to be wary of early discussion of consequences because this can be perceived as being punitive. Nurse managers should be business-like in their dealings with the aggressor. Heightened emotions and verbal retaliation should be scrupulously avoided—lest they trigger a return to an earlier phase of the cycle.

5. Post-crisis depression

The aggressor might experience depression, exhaustion, and remorse. These conditions might, in themselves, compromise the delivery of health care. Staff members need to judge when the time is most propitious to take the aggressor through an analysis of the antecedents, the person's behaviour, and the consequences of the hostile act. This analysis affords everyone an opportunity to identify and correct misunderstandings, identify and address inappropriate behaviours, and plan future safe contacts.

It is almost certain that staff members who are victims of significant aggression will exhibit diminished work performance in the short term. As a matter of urgency they should be replaced on their shift. Procedures for providing debriefing opportunities must be set in train. It is essential that all episodes of significant aggression be reported as *staff* incidents, as well as *patient* incidents.

> 'It is essential that all episodes of significant aggression be reported as *staff* incidents, as well as *patient* incidents.'

Conclusion

Aggression and hostility towards staff are endemic in healthcare systems around the globe. There is also an increase in hostility felt by overworked and highly stressed nursing staff towards their managers and coworkers. It is the responsibility of the nurse manager to have systems in place to deal with these scenarios. Policies and procedures should address issues of staff training in early identification of (and intervention for) aggression, organisational responses to unacceptable patient behaviour, and the provision of assistance to staff victims of aggression.

Aggression and hostility cannot be removed from the workplace because the intimate nature of healthcare delivery and the reality of human frailty mean that anxiety, fear, and misunderstanding will always be present. However, appropriate individual and organisational strategies will decrease the frequency of aggressive and hostile incidents.

Chapter 21

Managing Relatives' Concerns

Andrew Crowther

Introduction

As consumers of health services have become more knowledgeable about their care and treatment, their expectations have risen. There has been a similar growth in the knowledge and expectations of the relatives of those receiving care—relatives want and expect higher standards of care and treatment. This chapter explores some of the background to relatives' concerns and suggests some strategies that can be used by nurse managers when meeting with a concerned relative.

The nature of concern

The increased knowledge of patients and relatives has heightened their expectations of hospitals, health services, and the staff of these organisations. Informed and empowered by a plethora of television dramas and 'reality' programs, relatives are increasingly seeking information about all aspects of treatment, and are expecting informed, reasoned answers. These questions, and the expectation of adequate replies, can become more pressing if the patient is paying for his or her own care. However, it is still not uncommon to encounter patients, and their relatives, who have unbounded confidence in the healthcare team and who accept, with implicit trust, whatever is done. The Box below lists some matters about which relatives often have concerns.

Relatives' concerns

Relatives' concerns commonly centre on:
- concern that the clinical care being given is of the highest quality;
- the nature of the illness;
- access to a second opinion;
- the treatment to be given;
- whether the patient will have to wait for treatment;
- whether the patient will suffer pain;
- whether alternative treatments have been considered;
- the expected outcome of the treatment;
- the duration of treatment;
- the prognosis (and, in the case of a poor prognosis, the probable course of the illness);
- the expected level of functioning upon recovery;
- the location of the patient's recovery (home or another care facility?); and
- (if the patient is to be nursed at home) the nature of the care and the identity of the caregiver.

Concerned relatives often want to know the answer to all of their questions at once. The questions should be answered by the appropriate members of the medical staff or clinical nursing staff. The few occasions on which the nurse manager should be directly involved are those in which a junior nurse has been unable to provide satisfactory answers to relatives' questions, or when relatives wish to make a complaint about care or the behaviour or attitude of a member of the nursing staff.

These concerns can become magnified in the presence of ventilators, monitors, and even the ubiquitous intravenous pump. Medical technology and a large number of nurses can markedly increase relatives' concerns and fears.

A similar situation can occur in mental-health areas, in which the sometimes intimidating care environment and the behaviour of patients can agitate relatives. In these situations relatives often have a strong wish not to go home and leave their loved one 'alone'. Relatives of 'detained' patients (also known in different jurisdictions as 'sectioned' or 'recommended' patients) also need to know the exact legal status of their next-of-kin, and when and how the detention is to be reviewed.

Irritation experienced by relatives is often compounded by the realities of the clinical care of the patient. Long periods of boredom sitting by the bed of a silent loved one are interspersed with requests to 'wait outside for a moment'—and these enforced absences from the patient's side can be frustrating and worrying. The situation is made worse if the reason for the temporary absence and a full explanation of what occurred during that absence are not provided. It is the responsibility of the nurse manager to ensure that staff members adequately deal with this aspect of care. Providing important information helps to decrease the level of concern being experienced by relatives.

> 'Providing important information helps to decrease the level of concern being experienced by relatives.'

Milieu

The atmosphere of the environment in which a patient is receiving care has a significant effect on the unease experienced by relatives. The *milieu* (French for 'in the midst') of the ward can be influenced by the nurse manager and the clinical team with the specific aim of ensuring a non-threatening, restful atmosphere. Contemporary hospital architects and design consultants have made significant changes to the way in which clinical areas are now decorated in an attempt to minimise the harshness of traditional hospital environments. This has been particularly effective in the design of clinical areas in which children receive care, and in some of the more carefully planned mental-health treatment facilities.

> 'The milieu of the ward can be influenced by the nurse manager and the clinical team to ensure a non-threatening, restful atmosphere.'

All clinical-care staff members, whatever their grade or speciality, have had personal experience of how challenging the first day of work in any clinical area can be. That first shift stays in the memory—feelings of awkwardness, of being the only one who does not know what to do, and the bustle and pressure of a busy ward all combine to induce a sense of unease and discomfort. As familiarity with the ward grows, the sense of strangeness dissipates, and the ward ceases to be an alien environment. Indeed, clinical staff members can become so comfortable with their work area that they begin to see it as 'the norm', and can express surprise that new staff members (or patients' relatives) might find the area hostile or threatening. Those first-day feelings are repeated, albeit to a progressively less-marked degree, as staff are rotated through different wards or different hospitals.

It is important that nurses remain aware of those first-day feelings of bewilderment and unease—for this is how the relatives of patients can feel when they first encounter an unfamiliar clinical environment. The strange and unknown can combine with a deep concern for ill loved ones—resulting in relatives feeling threatened and vulnerable. This sense of threat and vulnerability can return if patients are transferred to another area, or are taken temporarily to another department for investigation or treatment.

> 'The strange and unknown can combine with a deep concern for ill loved ones—resulting in relatives feeling threatened and vulnerable.'

Other aspects of the ward or clinical activity can also impact on relatives' experiences of that area. These include the way in which staff members communicate with each other (particularly if abrupt, harsh, or demeaning language is used), the way in which the ward comes to a tense standstill when a chief executive or other senior person arrives, the reactions of staff members who do not feel valued by the manager, and the effects on staff dynamics if a nurse comes on duty late. If these behaviours are compounded by a death in the treatment area or a flurry of new admissions, relatives' experiences become significantly more stressful and unpleasant.

It is therefore important that the nurse manager ensures that staff members meet the needs of relatives adequately. This involves the nurse manager working with the clinical staff to ensure that relatives are not seen as nuisances who get in the way of nurses doing their work. Rather, relatives should be viewed as people with vital roles to play as partners in the care of patients. This can be achieved by establishing a *relatives' protocol* to be followed by all staff members. Such a protocol can alleviate relatives' concerns by ensuring that they receive an

> 'Relatives are not nuisances who get in the way of nurses doing their work . . . they are people with vital roles to play as partners in the care of patients.'

introduction to the primary nurse, a tour of the ward, and information about the location of cafés, outdoor sitting areas, and so on.

Changing information needs

As sick patients improve, the information needs of relatives change. Earlier concern for their loved ones and a desire for their speedy return to health are replaced by other concerns as patients improve, and both patients and relatives can become more demanding. In some countries and states concern might be expressed about the cost of the treatment. This concern can extend to worry about the indirect costs of a hospital admission—such as travelling to and from the hospital, accommodation and childcare costs, and so on. Possible loss of earnings, both for the patient and relatives, can also be a significant issue.

Attention can also turn to such seemingly insignificant matters as the type and décor of the patient's room, poor reception on the television set, problems with a snoring neighbour, or the punctuality of meals. This is not surprising because relatives suddenly find that their concern and attention are now less required by their loved ones. Relatives now need to redirect (or displace) these emotions onto something else. The nurse manager is likely to become involved in these instances. As concern for patients dissipates and concern becomes attached to other things—matters that might seem insignificant to nurses on the ward—the irritation of relatives can increase, and a more senior nurse might be required to address relatives' concerns.

> 'As concern for patients dissipates, concern becomes attached to other things—matters that might seem insignificant to nurses on the ward.'

Wider concerns

As ill patients recover, relatives can become increasingly preoccupied with wider issues—such as perceived care problems likely to occur after discharge of the patient, other long-standing (perhaps untreated) medical problems, housing, bullying at school, paying bills, and so on.

Attention thus moves from critically ill patients to recovering patients who are soon to go home, and relatives become concerned about the problems that recovering patients are likely to face. Depending upon organisational protocols and practices in a particular situation, these issues might fall within the remit of the ward team, or the nurse manager might need to become involved.

Community settings

The nurse manager of a team based in the community has slightly different problems and concerns with which to deal. In these situations, relatives have more power. The care setting might be the relative's home, and the nurse–relative relationship is thus reversed in terms of familiarity with the environment and control of activities in that environment. From the relative's perspective, there is often a lesser focus on the environment in which the patient receives care, and a greater focus on the frequency and quality of visits by the care team.

'In community settings relatives have more power . . . the nurse–relative relationship is reversed in terms of familiarity with the environment and control of activities.'

In this situation the nurse manager is unlikely to become involved with relatives' concerns unless there has been a significant problem with the nurse, the patient, or the relative during care delivery.

Patient liaison officers

In some larger health services and hospitals a *patient liaison officer* (sometimes called a 'complaints officer') is employed. Such a person should be the first point of contact for concerned relatives because such officers are likely to have expertise in dealing with distressed or truculent relatives.

The patient liaison officer is usually located in a private area, away from the bustle of the ward, and is thus able to engage in a confidential and private interview. These members of the healthcare team offer a very effective link for relatives who are bewildered by a complex and alien hospital environment.

Patient liaison officers are perceived as being very much 'on the side' of the patient and next-of-kin, and as being a friendly face in a sea of hurrying, busy health professionals. However, many hospitals that are fortunate enough to employ such an officer cannot stretch the budget to cover evening or weekend shifts. In these circumstances, if a problem arises that would normally have been dealt with by a patient liaison officer, the nurse manager could well become involved.

Strategies for nurse managers

It can be difficult for nurse managers to make time in busy shifts to spend time with concerned relatives, but it is important that they do so. It should be remembered that a nurse manager can appear to relatives to be an intimidating person, retaining much of the 'power figure' persona with which matrons and assistant matrons were endowed in past decades. Uniforms, pagers, and mobile phones can increase this perception. This can mean that concerned relatives, intimidated by an atmosphere of urgency and activity, might not persist with their requests to see someone—believing that the manager is too busy to bother with their apparently petty problems. Nonetheless, finding the time and a place

> 'It should be remembered that a nurse manager can appear to be an intimidating person . . . who is too busy to bother with relatives' apparently petty problems.'

to spend time with concerned relatives is a vital function of the nurse manager, and one that should not be put off.

If possible, any interview should occur away from ward noise, and the possibility of being overheard. If the relative wishes to have the patient present, this should be respected. Conversely, if the relative wishes to discuss matters in the absence of the patient, this should also be respected. In either case, permission to discuss the patient should always be obtained from the patient. An open-ended question (along the lines of: 'Is it OK to talk in front of your father or . . . ?') will usually suffice.

If the relative is truculent or loud, or gives any other cause for concern, the nurse manager should have another staff member present, and should sit between the relative and the door. All protocols with respect to duress alarms and the possibility of needing to summon assistance should be adhered to. If possible, pagers, mobile phones, and the like should be switched off or left with another person. The nurse manager should state how much time he or she has available for the interview, sit on the same level as the relative, and then actively listen. Being calm and speaking in a quiet, even voice will set the tone for the interview. Part of the role of the nurse manager, albeit an unwelcome one, is to absorb anger on behalf of the care team. Sitting and listening, and interjecting the occasional word of encouragement or understanding, can accomplish this. Often the burning issue that preoccupies the relative will diminish as the anger itself diminishes, and a calm exploration of the issue can then take place.

It is important that the nurse manager does more than simply pay attention to the relative during the interview. It can take courage for a relative to speak with a nurse manager, and that courage must be rewarded by more than a vague promise to 'look into it' or to 'see what can be done'. Details of what is going to occur must be shared with the relative. This applies whether the nurse manager is going to speak to the treating doctor, discuss options with the ward nurse, expedite a patient transfer, or follow an issue up with hospital services. It is vital that the relative knows what is happening at all times.

Strategies for nurse managers

In conducting an interview with concerned relatives, especially those who are agitated or truculent, nurse managers should keep the following strategies in mind:
- in the midst of a busy day, recognise the importance of relatives' concerns, and find the time and place to attend to those concerns;
- ensure privacy for the relatives and consent from the patient;
- if the relative is truculent, have another staff member present, follow all protocols with respect to duress alarms and the possibility of needing to summon assistance, remain calm, and attempt to diminish anger;
- ensure that the relative knows what is happening at all times with respect to follow up;
- establish a timeframe for follow up actions and ensure that it is kept;
- ensure that relatives are fully aware of the name and contact details of any other staff member who is given responsibility for resolving the matters causing concern;
- be aware of any stipulated mandatory reporting requirements and follow all protocols; and
- document the interview as appropriate.

All of these matters are discussed in this section of the chapter.

A timeframe must be put on the actions to follow the interview. Trust between the relative and nurse manager is engendered if the nurse manager states where, when, and how he or she will get back to the concerned relative and share the outcomes of any action. Establishing a definite timeframe also demonstrates the value of the relative consulting the nurse manager in the first instance.

'Trust is engendered if the nurse manager states where, when, and how he or she will get back to the concerned relative and share the outcomes of any action.'

If a sudden increase in workload, sick leave, or other unforeseen circumstances makes it impossible for the nurse manager to keep to the agreed timeframe and arrangements for follow-up, this should be communicated to the relative as soon as possible. Failure to do so decreases trust and respect, and can harm the image of the nurse manager and the employer.

If the nurse manager decides to refer any matter to another manager or employee, this decision must also be communicated to the relative. To enable the relative to follow up the issue appropriately, the contact details of the new person involved should also be provided.

The nurse manager should also be aware of any stipulated mandatory reporting that applies in the jurisdiction in which he or she works, and should follow protocols as necessary.

It is not advisable to make notes as an interview progresses. However, as with all other interventions, early documentation is important. Soon after the interview has finished, the discussion and its outcomes should be documented. Depending on the circumstances and the hospital or health service policies, a copy of the documentation might be given to the relative.

> 'Soon after the interview has finished, the discussion and its outcomes should be documented.'

Feedback

As hospitals and health services increasingly focus on measurement of service outcomes, there is a growing tendency to offer relatives some form of 'satisfaction survey' or 'outcome measurement tool'. These cover various aspects of the care and treatment of patients, as well as relatives' perceptions of their own experiences—such as whether they were greeted, whether they were kept informed, and whether they felt involved in decisions regarding care and treatment.

Such tools are very useful to the nurse manager. A clear picture can be gained of the service's strengths and weaknesses with respect to liaison with relatives and the skill levels of specific staff members. Nursing staff can receive praise as appropriate, and modifications can be made to the manner in which relatives are involved in the care of patients.

Conclusion

Contemporary health care is characterised by an ever-increasing awareness on the part of both patients and relatives of the standards of care that should be provided by hospitals and health services. These increased expectations have added another level of complexity to the role of the nurse manager. However, at the same time, they provide opportunities for service improvement and staff development.

'Increased expectations provide opportunities for service improvement and staff development.'

Chapter 22

Evidence-based Management

Peter French

Introduction

The application of evidence-based practice to healthcare management is relevant to all people in all levels of health care—especially the nurse manager, whose responsibility is the overall coordination of the nursing team.

Management, health care, and the evidence base

The term *management* assumes the existence of a large organisation that devotes resources to a particular purpose in society. In this case, the particular purpose in society is *health care* (includes primary, secondary, and tertiary healthcare activities). The *evidence base* includes both what the evidence is, and how it is conceived as evidence.

Taken together, this implies that evidence-based management (EBM) involves a proactive search for all available evidence, and that ignorance of the available knowledge will result in decisions that are less efficient (or at least less informed). In short, evidence produces decision-making for best practice in the management function in question. Management decisions are therefore not based on historical precedent; nor are they based on instinct or how a senior manager thinks things should be done. Rather, decision-making should be based on available evidence on best practice.

Organisational management

The processes of setting and achieving goals, as well as the coordination of information, are especially relevant to the concept of evidence-based healthcare management. The main roles of the manager are interpersonal, informational, and decisional in nature (Lussier 2003; Plunkett, Attner & Allen 2002). Two of these—informational and decisional—are closely implicated in evidence-based management.

Health care

Health care is primarily concerned with the maximisation of the health of society. Health care is not simply a matter of 'caring' in the emotional or altruistic sense. The healthcare industry is also concerned with politics and economics. The emerging need for evidence to substantiate practice is largely due to the increasing complexity of this interface.

> 'Health care is not simply a matter of 'caring' in the emotional or altruistic sense . . . it is also concerned with politics and economics.'

This chapter discusses some of the contemporary management issues that give rise to the emergence of evidence-based decision-making, before addressing the practical aspects of collating and evaluating the evidence.

EBM in the technological age

The ability to manage information is becoming more crucial. New technologies have brought about dramatic economies of scale. Much of the available information has been coordinated on and by the world-wide web, and this has accelerated the production of new information. To cope with this explosion in information, there has been a commensurate emergence of increasingly sophisticated information technology to access and organise information.

A major element of effective evidence-based practice is the ability to filter information that is not meaningful or understandable. This is the primary reason for the existence of the *systematic review* as the beginning of the process of evidence-based practice.

Human information-processing and decision-making

> This tendency of human minds to construct concepts is linked to biological and social survival; it allows human agents to recognize the same or similar stimuli when they are next encountered . . . By planning and executing the appropriate response to the stimulus, they render their worlds manageable.
>
> GREENWOOD (1996)

The decisions that are made, and the actions that are implemented, are determined by what a nurse manager *thinks*. Decision-making is a process of inductive reasoning that requires the selection of one option from a number of alternatives. Decision-making can thus be understood as an exercise in information-processing. This approach models thinking in terms of a number of stages—with each stage being a level of modification of an information input. Information-processing models examine the quality, quantity, and nature of the information, the stages of processing, and the outcome. An early information-processing model of decision-making (Gelatt 1962) has been adopted in research on the patient-centredness of nurses' decisions (French 1999).

The management of change

Change is an important issue in EBM simply because evidence-based practice can be viewed as a *change process*.

EBM sees change as a 'constant'. However, the direction of change and the acceleration of some aspects of change can be influenced by accurate information—or, in other words, 'evidence' that supports suppositions, decisions, policies, and practices.

Managed care

It has been said that the current global challenge in health care is the development of market-based competition (Buerhaus 1998). Economic forces are steadily taking priority over social welfare and professional imperatives in driving healthcare systems. Transformations are therefore taking place in the way that care is delivered. As employers seek lower costs and efficient services, managed care organisations are emerging in many countries—which respond to these demands by passing some of the pressure of resource allocation onto insurance companies, hospitals, and other contracting healthcare providers (Buerhaus 1998).

In this setting, the objective of the healthcare manager in delivering healthcare interventions is *not* to deliver *as much as possible* within a desired budget. Rather, it is to decide on *which* healthcare interventions to adopt. These must be chosen with a view to producing the greatest benefit to patients (or to do the least harm to patients). Information is thus required so that decisions can be made as to what investigations and interventions can be provided within a given economic climate. In some cases, this involves *generating* resources, as well as *using* them appropriately.

> 'The objective is not to deliver as much as possible within a desired budget. Rather, it is to decide on *which* healthcare interventions to adopt.'

Many aspects of 'managed care' are filtering into healthcare organisations that are not strictly 'managed-care organisations' in the usual sense of that term. Benefits emerge in the form of: (i) improved treatment outcomes; (ii) enhanced quality-of-life indicators; (iii) improved patient satisfaction; (iv) decreased mortality; (v) shorter length of stay; (vi) decreased re-admission rates; and (vii) lower relapse rates. The implementation processes for achieving acceptable cost/benefit ratios in these outcomes are: (i) standards for practice; (ii) clinical guidelines; (iii) performance indicators; and (iv) benchmarking.

These transformations in the management-value system have also been brought about by an increase in public accountability. This has brought about an increasing public and political interest in the evidence on which decisions about the effectiveness and safety of health care are based (Gray 1997).

Case management and the need for evidence

At the practitioner level, terms such as *evidence-based medicine* and *evidence-based nursing* are used. One process by which the two are brought closely together is through the use of information systems (related to case management) that have been designed largely to provide openness and accountability. To utilise evidence, the organisation needs to be able to (Matthews 2002):

▶ gain access to data in a timely manner;
▶ maintain the quality and integrity of the data (and thus confidence in that data);
▶ identify the data source;

▶ acknowledge clear ownership of the data;
▶ integrate data across the patient care continuum and across multiple organisations and practitioners;
▶ obtain compliance, regulatory, and accreditation support; and
▶ provide patient confidentiality and security.

Managed care

Benefits
The benefits of managed care are:
* improved treatment outcomes;
* enhanced quality-of-life indicators;
* improved patient satisfaction;
* decreased mortality;
* shorter length of stay;
* decreased re-admission rates; and
* lower relapse rates.

Implementation processes
The implementation processes for achieving acceptable cost/benefit ratios in these outcomes are:
* standards for practice;
* clinical guidelines;
* performance indicators; and
* benchmarking.

Evidence-based practice

There are several different dimensions to the concept of evidence-based practice (French 2002):
▶ the *datum* dimension—research findings *vs* any relevant information;
▶ the *scientific* dimension—inclusion of interpretive approaches *vs* the exclusion of those approaches;
▶ the *social* dimension—the individual patient *vs* patient group focus; and
▶ the *organisational* dimension—individual practitioner *vs* organisational decision-making.

It was has also been concluded there are several concomitants of evidence-based practice. They are (French 2002):
▶ information management;
▶ clinical judgment and problem-solving;

‣ professional practice development;
‣ managed care; and
‣ research findings.

Although there is no single meaning of the term 'evidence', each organisation will come up with its own fairly pragmatic definition of evidence-based practice (EBP).

Identifying EBM issues

The process of evidence-based healthcare management is about *consensual* decision-making; it is *not* a process for nurse managers working in isolation. From the earliest stages, the relevance and appropriateness of evidence-based decisions must be decided.

There are several ways in which this can be done. The most important issue in this process is consensual agreement. This is best achieved by use of one or more of the following:

‣ quality circles;
‣ nominal-group technique;
‣ the Delphi process; and
‣ top–down decisions.

Each of these is discussed below.

Quality circles

Quality circles (QCs) consist of small groups of people from the same or similar work units who voluntarily meet to identify and analyse problems, and to recommend solutions to their work-related problems.

Quality circles can sometimes be ineffective because members of the circle are often very senior, and the autocratic behaviour of some members can stifle open debate. In addition, if there is no real apparent progress made, members often find QCs meaningless as time goes by. Insult is added to injury if staff are repeatedly taken away from clinical commitments.

'The autocratic behaviour of some members can stifle open debate.'

These obstacles must be considered before QCs are adopted as a forum for identifying evidence-based healthcare management issues. The requirements for an efficient and productive QC are:

‣ organisational support;
‣ open access for all staff;

▶ inputs of informed opinion;
▶ achievement of group consensus;
▶ follow-up action; and
▶ steering and monitoring of implementation by the QC.

Consensual decision-making

Consensual agreement is best achieved by use of one or more of the following:
- quality circles;
- nominal-group technique;
- the Delphi process; and
- top–down decisions.

  Each of these is discussed in this section of the text.

The nominal-group technique

The nominal-group technique is a method for structuring a group communication process so that it is effective in allowing a group of individuals to deal with a complex problem (Linstone & Turoff 1975). This process gathers opinions from a relatively small group of people who can meet face to face (Delbecq, Van de Ven & Gustafson 1975). Consensus is achieved by facilitating equal input from every individual in the group.

'Consensus is achieved by facilitating equal input from every individual in the group.'

Essentially the following steps occur.

▶ The question is specified. Individuals independently generate answers to the question. All suggestions are collated on one display visible to the whole group, and are *not* changed or rejected by the facilitator.
▶ Duplicate suggestions are removed by group discussion. If there is lack of consensus or a reasonable doubt, the suggestions are preserved.
▶ Each item is given a code number or letter for ease of reference.
▶ Each member then selects 3–5 responses that he or she thinks are most relevant to the question. The scores of each member are then recorded on the group display and the items receiving the most 'marks' are identified and ranked.
▶ Discussion then takes place on the meaning of the results.

  This process works best with groups of approximately 15–30 people, and takes approximately 2–3 hours. One of the benefits of this process is that group

> 'The focus is not on what the manager knows, but on what the manager does not yet know.'

members contribute vocally *and* physically. The process also minimises the influence of individuals who dominate committee meetings. In addition, a process of creative thinking is facilitated, and sometimes the most unexpected trains of thought result in a surprise solution. The nominal-group process is highly effective because the focus is not on what the manager (or participant) knows, but on what the manager (or participant) does not yet know.

The Delphi process

The Delphi process has many similarities to the nominal-group technique, but is conducted with a larger number of people who are not able to come together in a face-to-face situation. A Delphi survey utilises a panel of 'experts' to obtain a consensus opinion on a complex matter (French, Ho & Lee 2002). One advantage of this method is that responses provide numerous examples of precise issues in the actual words of the respondents. A prioritised list produced in this way provides data that are useful in the decision-making process, but it does not provide a ready-made answer. It is still the responsibility of the quality circle or management group to delimit each quality-of-care issue.

One way of achieving this is to structure quality circles as evidence-based decision-making groups.

Top–down decisions

Executives, bosses, and boards often develop their own personal issues that are amenable to evidence-based approaches. In some cases, organisations have certain traditions, or are preoccupied with certain historical issues. At a more objective level, research reports, consultant evaluations, market research, or government inquiries can indicate problems that are amenable to evidence-based processes.

The systematic review

However the problems are identified, the EBM approach assumes that accurate evidence is required, and that this evidence should be collected and systematically evaluated. The process that is most commonly used for this evaluation is the *systematic review*.

Systematic review, together with *meta-analysis*, comprises what is now called 'secondary research'. This consists of the analysis and synthesis of the findings of primary research papers to produce a conclusion on the state of the knowledge base on a particular problem.

Meta-analysis tends to aggregate the data from replicated studies. It has been said that 'reviews should be held to the same standards of clarity, methodology, and replication as primary research' (Ganong 1987, p. 2). These reviews should be explicit about the process adopted, and there should be sufficient information to allow readers of the review to judge the quality of the findings of that review (Gray 1997). Such a review should be:

▶ comprehensive—covering all available related knowledge;
▶ relevant—focused on a specific and operationalised problem;
▶ objective—impartial and subject to independent confirmation;
▶ critical—utilising cognitive skills to make judgments;
▶ methodical—using tried-and-tested (and explicit) processes;
▶ open to analysis and the judgment of others;
▶ accountable—explaining the strengths and weaknesses of the review; and
▶ responsible—having a commitment to update the review frequently (for example, every 2–3 years).

The process of review involves six tasks (Jackson 1980):

▶ selecting the question for review;
▶ sampling the research to be reviewed;
▶ representing the characteristics of the studies and their findings;
▶ analysing findings;
▶ interpreting the results; and
▶ reporting the review.

The more important of these steps are discussed in further detail below.

Selecting the question for review

The formulation of this question has a very influential effect on the selection of the problem, the efficiency of the review process, and the outcome. There will always be variations in terminology, back-tracking, and reformulation of ideas.

The reviewer should not take this stage of the review process for granted, and should consciously reflect on the choices made and be able to explain them to others. The number of questions increases the workload by multiples of the original question. It is easy to generate

'It is easy to generate questions, but not easy to be decisive and select the best option that will produce the best results.'

questions, but not easy to be decisive and select the best option that will produce the best results for a management decision.

Sampling the research to be reviewed

The first step is the search using the critical *key words*. These key words are essentially the concepts that target the key components of the issue or problem. This process of selection of key words requires an understanding of the core concept and the different words that might be used to describe it. Labels for concepts can be subject to changes in knowledge (and changes in fashion).

Databases can consist of traditional library holdings—such as books, theses, dissertations, journals, newspapers, and reports. Accessing these holdings is usually achieved by searching index lists that state the title, authors, and time and place of the publication. These individual references are often accompanied by shorter abstracts (usually limited to approximately 300 words). These enable the reader to make a quick judgment as to the relevance of the paper.

Much of the process of indexing and making available abstracts has been transformed into electronic databases—such as MEDLINE and CINAHL.

The systematic review

The process of systematic review involves six tasks:
- selecting the question for review;
- sampling the research to be reviewed;
- representing the characteristics of the studies and their findings;
- analysing findings;
- interpreting the results; and
- reporting the review.

The more important of these steps are discussed in further detail in this section of the text.

Adapted from Jackson (1980)

Analysing findings and interpreting results

To evaluate the composite research findings and results, two estimates should be taken. The first is to estimate the validity and reliability of the *findings*, and the second is to estimate the validity and reliability of the *recommendations*.

Consideration should be given to:
- designs;
- samples;

➧ measures; and

➧ findings.

Designs should also be considered in terms of their diversity. This should not be too difficult if the process of inclusion and exclusion specifies designs of a particular type (for example, experimental or survey).

Samples should also be considered in terms of the diversity of subjects in different studies, and the specification of the sampling procedure.

Summarising the *measures* and the *findings* requires an assessment of the statistical effectiveness of the type of data, together with an assessment of the appropriateness and reliability of the measure that was used. Similarly, consideration should be given to the appropriateness of the analytical procedure and the degree to which the findings for the sample can be said to reflect the parameters of the wider population.

Once the *findings* have been assessed for validity and reliability, the validity of *recommendations* can be assessed by asking the following questions.

➧ Are the systematic review findings directly related to the review question?

➧ Are the recommendations directly derived from the findings?

➧ Did the recommendations consider all the structural, process, and outcome elements of the situation?

➧ Are there success criteria specified for outcomes?

➧ Are the recommendations evaluated and prioritised by the authors?

In a clinical area, the effectiveness of recommendations can be assessed by asking the following questions.

➧ What is the degree of uncertainty associated with the findings?

➧ What are the benefits and advantages to patients?

➧ What are the outcomes and risks for patients?

➧ What is the impact of clinician preferences?

➧ What is the impact of patient preferences?

➧ What influence has the cost/benefit equation imposed by the institution?

➧ Are there differences in any of these things associated with different client groups?

Implementing best practice: action research

The processes that have been outlined above give an overview of the most important points to consider when preparing a systematic review. Once the review is prepared, the best form of implementation should be considered.

In many healthcare management situations, the main consideration is not what should be done, but how confident the manager can be that practices reported elsewhere are better than those currently in place. There is often a dilemma in management about the implementation of new practices based on evidence that has been collected in a different context from the one in which it will be applied (French 2000).

The following sorts of questions present themselves.

▶ Will the practice have any unforeseen disadvantages in the new situation?
▶ How can we make sure that the situation does not become worse?

The implementation of new practices must be carefully monitored so that risks can be carefully managed. *Action research* is ideal for this purpose. However, it is rarely adopted as a process for monitoring change.

Action research is the design and refinement of a process of social change by engaging in cycles of data-collection and decision-making along with the people who are part of the change process (Lewin 1947). Four conditions for action research have been described. The conditions are (Carr & Kemis 1986):

▶ that the subject matter is a social practice;
▶ that change in practice is necessary and can be objectified;
▶ that the project proceeds through a number of cycles of planning, acting, observing, and reflecting; and
▶ that the project involves all who are responsible for the practice in each of the moments of the activity.

During action research, the social change must be objectified in the form of a guideline, procedure, or protocol. The best data-collection methods are then selected with a view to selecting those that help the team to understand the effectiveness of the new process. All participants in the change setting (patients, staff, family) provide data, and they participate in the interpretation of the analysed data. They also subsequently suggest improvements in the guidelines that control the newly implemented activity.

This cycle of events is continued (daily, weekly, or monthly) until the best and most efficient guideline for the change has been produced to the satisfaction of all participants. Because data-collection and decision-making cycles follow a tight timetable, dangers and unacceptable risks can be identified quickly, and measures can be taken to prevent any harm that occurs.

Conclusion

As in all other aspects of nursing, there is an increasingly urgent need for nursing-management practices to be firmly based on reliable evidence if the strategies that are adopted are to have the desired outcome. The processes by which evidence-based management are established mimic those adopted in clinical areas. An understanding of these techniques is essential for the contemporary nurse manager.

References

Chapter 1 The Nurse Manager

Duffield, C., Moran, P., Beutel, J., Bunt, S., Thornton, A., Wills, J., Cahill, P. & Franks, H. 2001, 'Profile of First-line Managers in New South Wales, Australia, in the 1990s', *Journal of Advanced Nursing*, vol. 36 no. 6, p. 786.

Goleman, D. 2000, 'Leadership that Gets Results', *Harvard Business Review*, March/April, p. 80.

Maccoby, M. 2001, 'The Human Side: Successful Leaders Employ Strategic Intelligence', *Research Technology Management*, May/June, pp 43–5.

RCNA *see* Royal College of Nursing, Australia.

Royal College of Nursing, Australia 2000, 'Australia's Position Statement on the Management of Nursing and Midwifery Services', RCNA.

Chapter 3

Beauchamp,T.L. & Childress, J.F. 2001, *Principles of Biomedical Ethics*, 5th edn, Oxford University Press, Oxford.

Berwick, D., Davidoff, F., Hiatt, H. & Smith, R. 2001, 'Refining and Implementing the Tavistock Principles for Everybody in Health Care, *British Medical Journal*, vol. 323, pp 616–19.

Canadian Nurses' Association 2000, *Working with Limited Resources: Nurses' Moral Constraints*, Author, Ottawa.

CNA, *see* Canadian Nurses' Association.

Chambliss, D.F. 1996, *Beyond Caring: Hospitals, Nurses, and the Social Organisation of Ethics*, The University of Chicago Press, Chicago.

ICN, *see* International Council of Nurses.

International Council of Nurses 2000, 'ICN Code of Ethics', available online at <www.icn.ch/ethics.htm>.

International Council of Nurses 2003, <www.icn.ch>.

Jameton, A. 1984, *Nursing Practice: The Ethical Issues*, Prentice-Hall, Englewood Cliffs, N.J..

Kelly, B. 1996, '"Hospital nursing: It's a battle!" A Follow-up Study of English Graduate Nurses', *Journal of Advanced Nursing*, 24(5), pp 1063–9.

Kelly, B. 1998, 'Preserving Moral Integrity: A Follow-up Study with New Graduate Nurses (experience before and throughout the nursing career)', *Journal of Advanced Nursing*, 28(5), pp 1134–45.

May, L. 1996, *The Socially Responsive Self: Social Theory and Professional Ethics*, The University of Chicago Press, Chicago.

Reiser, S. 1994, 'The Ethical Life of Health Care Organizations', *Hastings Centre Report*, 24, no. 6.

Secker, B. 2002, personal correspondence, University of Toronto Joint Centre for Bioethics, Toronto.

Webster, G.C. & Baylis, F. 2000, 'Moral Residue' in S.B. Rubin & L. Zoloth (eds), *Margin of Error: The Ethics of Mistakes in the Practice of Medicine*, University Publishing Group, Hagerstown, MD.

Chapter 4 Leading, Motivating, and Enthusing

Adair, J. 1983, *Effective Leadership*, Gower, London.

Falcone, P. 2002, 'Motivating Staff Without Money', *HR Magazine*, August, pp 105–8.

Fiedler, F. & Chemers, M. 1974, *Leadership and Effective Management*, Scott Foresman, Illinois.
Fister-Gale, S. 2002, 'Building Leaders at All Levels', *Workforce*, October, 82–5.
Hall, P. 2002, 'How to Grow Your Own Leaders', *People Management*, June, 56–7.
Handy, C. 1999, *Understanding Organisations*, 4th edn, Penguin Books, London.
Henderson, E., Phillips, K. & Lewis, P. 2000, *Management in Health and Social Care: Understanding People*, *Module 2*, The Open University, Milton Keyes.
Hersey, P. & Blanchard, K.H. 1993, *Management of Organisational Behaviour: Utilizing Human Resources*, 6th edn, Prentice Hall, New Jersey.
House, R.J. 1971, 'A Path Goal Theory of Leader Effectiveness', *Administrative Science Quarterly*, 16(3), 321.
Kosinska, M. & Niebroj, L. 2003, 'The Position of a Leader Nurse', *Journal of Nursing Management*, 11, 69–72.
Maslow, A.H. 1970, *Motivation and Personality*, Harper & Row, New York.
McGregor, D. 1960, *The Human Side of Enterprise*, McGraw-Hill, New York.
Neisloss, S. 2002, '10 Steps to Better Credibility', *Pharmaceutical Executive*, December, 76–7.
Owen, H. 1990, *Leadership Is*, Abbot Publishing, Maryland.
Tappen, R. 2001, *Nursing Leadership & Management: Concepts and Practice*, 4th edn, F.A. Davis Company, Philadelphia.
Thyer, G. 2003, 'Dare to be Different: Transformational Leadership May Hold the Key to Reducing the Nursing Shortage', *Journal of Nursing Management*, 11, 73–9.
Trofino, A. 2000, 'Transformational Leadership: Moving Total Quality Management to World-Class Organisations', *International Nursing Review*, 47, 232–42.
Wright, S. 1993, 'The Standard Guide to Achieving Change Quietly', *Nursing Standard*, March, 7(26), 52–5.

Chapter 5 Working with Other Disciplines

Antonovsky, A. 1979, *Health, Stress and Coping*, Jossey-Bass, San Francisco.
Antonovsky, A. 1987, *Unraveling the Mysteries of Health: How People Manage Stress and Stay Well*, Jossey-Bass, San Francisco.
Kenny, G. 2002, 'Interprofessional Working: Opportunities and Challenges', *Nursing Standard*, 17(6): 33–5.
Scholes, J. & Vaughan, B. 2002, 'Cross-boundary Working: Implications for the Multiprofessional Team', *Journal of Clinical Nursing*, 11: 399–408.
Stuhlmiller, C.M. 1994, 'Rescuers of Cypress: Work Meanings and Practices that Guided Appraisal and Coping', *Western Journal of Nursing Research*, 16 (3): 268–87.
Stuhlmiller, C.M. 1996, *Rescuers of Cypress: Learning from Disaster* (Book 2 of the International Healthcare Ethics Series), Peter Lang Publishing, New York.
Stuhlmiller, C.M. 2000, 'Saluting Health', in Horsfall, J. & Stuhlmiller, C., *Interpersonal Nursing for Mental Health*, MacLennan & Petty, Sydney.
Stuhlmiller, C.M. 2003, 'Nurse–Consumer Collaboration: Go with the Flo!', in Barker, P., *Psychiatric and Mental Health Nursing* (Chapter 66), Arnold, London.
Taylor, B. 1994, *Being Human: Ordinariness in Nursing*, Churchill Livingstone, Melbourne.
West, E. & Scott, C. 2000, 'Nursing in the Public Sphere: Breaching the Boundary between Research and Policy', *Journal of Advanced Nursing*, 32(4): 817–24.

Chapter 6 Making Meetings Work

Chang, A. 1992, 'Conducting Conference Calls', *Association Management*, January: L55–L56, L78.
Constitution Society 2003, <www.constitution.org>.
Denholm, B. 1998, 'Parliamentary Procedure Promotes Order Out of Chaos', *AORN Journal*, March, vol. 67, no. 3, pp 590–600.
Hindle, T. 1998, *Managing Meetings*, DK Publishing, Inc., New York.
Nichols, G. 1998, 'How to Improve the Quality of the Meeting Process', *Association Management*, January: 74.
Partridge, W. 2000, 'Getting the Board to Measure Up', *Association Management*, January: 59–62.
Rogers, C. 1993, 'A Delegate's Guide to Parliamentary Law or How to Expedite Business Ensuring Justice, Equality, Order', *AORN Journal*, January, vol. 57, no. 1, pp 103–13.
Schlegel, J. 1994, 'Meaningful Meetings', *Association Management*, January: L46–L47.
Schlegel, J. 2000, 'Making Meetings Effective', *Association Management*, January, 121–2.

Chapter 7 Counselling Your Staff

Egan, G. 1998, *The Skilled Helper: A Problem-Management Approach to Helping*, 6th edn, Brooks Cole, Pacific Grove.

Geldard, D. & Geldard, K. 2001, *Basic Personal Counselling, a Training Manual for Counsellors*, 4th edn, Prentice Hall, Frenchs Forest.

Chapter 8 Dealing with Unhelpful Nurses

Archer, D. 1999, 'Exploring "bullying" culture in the para-military organisation', *International Journal of Manpower*, vol. 20 (1/2), pp 94–105.

Christie, B. & Kleiner, B.H. 2000, 'When is an Employee Unsalvageable?' *Equal Opportunities International*, vol. 19 (6/7), pp 40–4.

Clarke, S. 2003, 'The Contemporary Workforce: Implications for Organisational Safety Culture', *Personnel Review*, vol. 32(1), pp 40–57.

Collis, G. 2001, 'Bullies Not Wanted: Recognising and Eliminating Workplace Bullying', <www.employeeombudsman.sa.gov.au>.

Crawford, N. 1999, 'Conundrums and Confusion in Organisations: the Etymology of the Word "Bully"', *International Journal of Manpower*, vol. 20 (1/2), pp 86–94.

Elangovan, A.R. 2002, 'Managerial Intervention in Disputes: the Role of Cognitive Biases and Heuristics', *Leadership & Organisation Development Journal*, vol. 23 (7), pp 390–9.

Field, T. 1999, 'Those Who Can, Do: Those Who Can't, Bully', <www.bulliesdownunder.com/Field.htm>.

Hannabuss, S. 1998, 'Bullying at Work', *Library Management*, vol. 19 (5), pp 304–10.

Jetson, S. & Associates 2003, *Thriving at the Expense of Others: Bullying at Work*, Mt Lawley, Author, Western Australia.

Johnson, P.R. & Indvik, J. 2001, 'Slings and Arrows of Rudeness: Incivility in the Workplace', *Journal of Management Development*, vol. 20 (8), pp 705–14.

Rees, W.D. 1997, 'The Disciplinary Pyramid and Its Importance', *Industrial and Commercial Training*, vol. 29 (1), pp 4–9.

Tversky, A. & Kahneman, D. 1982, 'Judgments under Uncertainty: Heuristics and Biases', in D. Kahneman, P. Slovic & A. Tversky (eds), *Judgment under Uncertainty: Heuristics and Biases*, pp 3–20, Cambridge University Press, New York.

Chapter 9 Managing Performance

Ainsworth, M., Smith, N. & Millership, A. 2002, *Managing Performance. Managing People. Understanding and Improving Team Performance*, Pearson Education, Australia.

Chapter 10 Managing Risk

Aiken, L., Clarke, S., Sloane, D., Sochalski, J. & Silber, J. 2002, 'Hospital Nurse Staffing and Patient Mortality, Nurse Burnout, and Job Satisfaction', *Journal of American Medical Association*, 288: 1987–93.

Benner, P., Sheets, V., Uris, P. Malloch, K., Schwed, K. & Jamison, D. 2002, 'Individual Practice and System Causes of Errors in Nursing: A Taxonomy', *Journal of Nursing Administration*, 32: 509–23.

Berwick, D. 1989, 'Continuous Improvement as an Ideal in Healthcare', *New England Journal of Medicine*, 320: 3–56.

Donaldson, L. & Muir Gray, J. 1998, 'Clinical Governance: a Quality Duty for Health Organisations', *Quality in Health Care*, 7 (suppl): S37–S44.

Hewett, D. 2001, 'Supporting Staff Involved in Serious Incidents and During Litigation', in C. Vincent, *Clinical Risk Management: Enhancing Patient Safety*, pp 481–95, BMJ Books, London.

Kohn, L.T., Corrigan, J.M. & Donaldson, M.F. (eds) 1999, *To Err is Human. Building a Safer Health System*, Institute of Medicine, National Academy Press, Washington, D.C.

Leape, L. 1994, 'Error in Medicine', *Journal of American Medical Association*, 272(23): 1851–7.

Meurier, C. 2000, 'Understanding the Nature of Errors in Nursing: Using a Model to Analyse Critical Incident Reports of Errors which had Resulted in an Adverse or Potentially Adverse Event', *Journal of Advanced Nursing*, 32(1): 202–7.

Needleman, J., Buerhaus, P., Mattke, S., Stewart, M. & Zelevinsky, K. 2002, 'Nurse-Staffing Levels and Quality of Care in Hospitals', *New England Journal of Medicine*, 346: 1415–22.

Reason, J. 1997, *Managing the Risks of Organisational Accidents*, Ashgate Publishing Limited, Hampshire.

Richmond, J. (ed.) 2001, *Nursing Documentation: Writing What We Do*, Ausmed Publications, Melbourne.

Standards Australia 1999, *Risk Management AS/NZS 4360:1999*, Sydney.

Vecchi, L. 2003, 'Summary of Health Service Reviews: Patient Safety and Clinical Governance', Peter MacCallum Cancer Centre, Melbourne.

Vincent, C. (ed.) 2001, *Clinical Risk Management: Enhancing Patient Safety*, BMJ Books, London.

Vincent, C., Young, M. & Phillips, A. 1994, 'Why Do People Sue Doctors? A Study of Patients and Relatives Taking Legal Action', *Lancet*, 343: 1609–13.

Chapter 11 Occupational Health and Safety

Health & Safety Executive 1998, *Successful Health & Safety Management*, HSE Books, Sudbury, Suffolk.

Robens (Lord) 1972, 'Report of the Committee on Safety and Health at Work' (Chairman Lord Robens), HMSO, 1972.

WorkSafe WA *see* WorkSafe Western Australia.

WorkSafe Western Australia 2003a, *Code of Practice: Workplace Violence*, <www.safetyline.wa.gov.au>.

WorkSafe Western Australia 2003b, *Guidance Note. Dealing with Workplace Bullying. A Guide for Employers*, <www.safetyline.wa.gov.au>.

Chapter 12 Maximising the Quality Factor

Berwick, D. 1996, 'A Primer on Leading the Improvement of Systems', *British Medical Journal*, 312: 619–22.

Brassard, M. & D. Ritter 1994, *The Memory Jogger 11: A Pocket Guide of Tools for Continuous Improvement and Effective Planning*, Goal/QPC, Salem.

Leape, L., Kabcenell, A., Ghandi, T., Carver, P., Nolan, T. & Berwick, D. 2000, 'Reducing Adverse Drug Events: Lessons from a Breakthrough Series Collaborative', *Journal of Quality Improvement*, 26(6): 321–31.

NSW Health 2002, *Easy Guide to Clinical Practice Improvement: a Guide for Healthcare Professionals*, NSW Health Department, Sydney.

Scally, G. & L. Donaldson 2001, 'Clinical Governance and the Drive for Quality Improvement in the New NHS in England', *British Medical Journal*, 317: 61–5.

Vincent, C., Young, M. & Phillips, A. 1994, 'Why Do People Sue Doctors? A Study of Patients and Relatives Taking Legal Action', *Lancet*, 343: 1609–13.

Chapter 13 Writing Policies and Procedures

Hogwood, B.W.& Gunn, L.A. 1984, *Policy Analysis for the Real World*, Oxford University Press, Oxford.

Chapter 15 Selecting, Recruiting, and Retaining Staff

Fitzgerald, D. 2002, 'Nursing Shortage: A Crisis for the Next Decade', *Contemporary Nurse*, vol. 13, issue 2/3.

Gordon, A. 2002, 'Success Story: No Nursing Shortage Here', Institute for Healthcare Improvement, <www.ihl.org>.

Chapter 16 Rostering

Bonner, R., Beaumont, R. & Smith, B. 1995a, 'Understanding Rostering Part 1: The Rights and Wrongs of Rostering', *Australian Nursing Journal*, 18(2): 17–19.

Bonner, R., Beaumont, R. & Smith, B., 1995b, 'Understanding Rostering Part 2: The Rights and Wrongs of Rostering', *Australian Nursing Journal*, 2(9): 28–31.

Fudge, L. 2001, 'Team-based Self Rostering', *British Journal of Peri-operative Nursing*, 11(7): 310–16.

Vetter, E., Felice, L. & Ingersoll, G. 2001, 'Self-scheduling and Staff Incentives: Meeting Patient Care Needs in a Neonatal Intensive Care Unit', *Critical Care Nurse*, 21(4): 52–9.

Chapter 17 Budgeting

Finkler, S.A. & Kovner, C.T. 2000, *Financial Management for Nurse Managers and Executives*, 2nd edn, W.B. Saunders & Co., USA.

Grohar-Murray, M.E. & DiCroce, H.R. 2003, *Leadership and Management in Nursing*, 3rd edn, Prentice Hall, USA.

Huber, D. 2000, *Leadership and Nursing Care Management*, 2nd edn, W.B. Saunders & Co., Philadelphia.

Marquis, B.L. & Huston, C.J. 2003, *Leadership Roles and Management Functions in Nursing: Theory and Application*, 4th edn, J.B. Lippincott, Philadelphia.

Marrelli, T.M. 1997, *The Nurse Manager's Survival Guide: Practical Answers to Everyday Problems*, 2nd edn, Mosby-Year Book Inc., USA.

Chapter 18 Managing Information

Collins, R. & McLaughlin, Y. 1996, *Effective Management*, 2nd edn, CCH Australia, Sydney.

Davidhizar, R. & Shearer, R. 1999, 'Worklife: Some E-Mail Don'ts for Nurse Managers', *Canadian Nurse*, 95(9): 47–8.

Fayol, H. 1916, *Industrial and General Administration*, Dunod, Paris.

Feldman, H.R. 2000, 'E-mail: Nemesis or Savior', *Nursing Leadership Forum*, 5(2): 39.

FitzHenry, F. 1998, 'Consider this . . . Nursing Administrators and Clinical Information Systems: Shaping the future', *Journal of Nursing Administration*, 28(11): 24, 38, 45.

Hughes, J.A. & Pakieser, R.A. 1999, 'Factors that Impact Nnurses' Use of Electronic Mail', *Computers in Nursing*, 17(6): 251–8.

Kaufman, M.L. & Paulanka, B.L. 1994, 'Nursing Information: Better Outcomes, Less Costs', *Seminars for Nurse Managers*, 2(2): 102–9.

Martinez, M.N. 1997, 'Human Resources. Usage Policy Clears the Air about E-Mail', *Balance*, 1(4): 18–9.

Mulligan, E. 1998, 'Protecting Patient Confidentiality in Hospitals', *Australian Health Review*, 21(3): 67–77.

Murchison, R.S. 1999, 'Technology: Nursing the System. Get Patient Information Anytime, Anywhere', *Nursing Management*, 30(5): 19–20.

O'Brien, J. 1999, *Management Information Systems: Managing Information Technology in the Internetworked Enterprise*, 4th edn, Irwin McGraw-Hill, Sydney.

Richards, J.A. 2001, 'Nursing within a Digital Society', *Canadian Nurse*, 97(10): 14–15.

Robbins, S. & Mukerji, D. 1994, *Managing Organisations: New Challenges and Perspectives*, 2nd edn, Prentice Hall, Sydney.

Simpson, R.L. 1997, 'Technology: Nursing the System. CIOs and Trends in Health Care Computing', *Nursing Management*, 28(9): 20–1.

Styffe, E.J. 1997, 'Privacy, Confidentiality, and Security in Clinical Information Systems: Dilemmas and Opportunities for the Nurse Executive', *Nursing Administration Quarterly*, 21(3): 21–8.

Tapp, A. 2001, 'On the Job Legal Matters. The Legal Risk of E-mail', *Canadian Nurse*, 97(3): 35–6.

Chapter 19 The Nurse Manager as Educator

Argyris, C. 1991, 'Teaching Smart People How to Learn', *Harvard Business Review*, May–June 1991, pp 99–108.

Argyris, C. 2000, *On Organisational Learning*, Blackwell, Oxford.

CDH, see Council of Deans and Heads of UK University Faculties for Nursing, Midwifery and Health Visiting.

Council of Deans and Heads of UK University Faculties for Nursing, Midwifery and Health Visiting 1999, 'Developing a Clinical Academic Career for Nurses and Midwives: A Consultation Paper', July 1999.

Department of Health (UK) 2003, <www.doh.gov.uk/workingtime/guidance.htm>.

DoH, see Department of Health (UK).

ENB, see English National Board for Nursing, Midwifery and Health Visiting.

English National Board for Nursing, Midwifery and Health Visiting 1995, unpublished report presented to ENB National Research Conference 1995 (authors Alan Myles & Sue Frost).

Entwhistle, N. 1996, *Styles of Learning and Teaching: An Integrative Outline of Educational Psychology for Students, Teachers and Lecturers*, David Fulton & Sons, London.

Komives, S. & Woodard, D. 1996, *Student Services*, 3rd edn, Jossey Bass.

Moss Kanter, R. 1990, *When Giants Learn to Dance: Mastering the Challenges of Strategy, Management and Careers in the 1990s*, Routledge, an imprint of Taylor & Francis Ltd.

NMC, see Nursing and Midwifery Council (UK).

Nursing and Midwifery Council (UK) 1993, 'The Future of Professional Practice and Education. Final Draft Report', published as Paper One, CC/93/12, London UKCC.

Owen, H. 2001, *Unleashing Leaders*, John Wiley & Sons, Chichester, New York.

Richards, R. 1997, 'Clinical Academic Careers: Report of an Independent Task Force Chaired by Sir Rex Richards', Committee of Vice-Chancellors and Principals of the Universities of the UK, London.

Stewart, T. 2003, *Intellectual Capital: The New Wealth of Organisations*, Nicholas Brearly Publishing, London.
Wedderburn Tate, C. 1999, *Leadership in Nursing*, Churchill Livingstone.

Chapter 20 Coping with Hostility

Allen, M.H., Currier, G.W., Hughes, D.H., Reyes-Harde, M. & Docherty, J.P. 2001, *The Expert Consensus Guideline Series: Treatment of Behavioural Emergencies*, Expert Knowledge Systems, White Plains, N.Y.
Appelbaum, P., Robbins, P. & Monahan, J. 2000, 'Violence and Delusions: Data from the MacArthur Violence Risk Assessment Study', *American Journal of Psychiatry*, 157, pp 566–72.
Bowie, V. 1989, *Coping with Violence: A Guide for the Human Services*, Karibuni Press, Sydney.
CDHA, *see* Commonwealth Department of Health and Ageing.
Central Sydney Area Health Service 2001, *Prevention and Management of Workplace Aggression: Guidelines and Case Studies from the NSW Health Industry*, Author, Sydney.
Commonwealth Department of Health and Ageing 2002, *Comorbidity of Mental Disorders and Substance Abuse: A Brief Guide for the Primary Care Clinician*, Author, Canberra.
CSAHS, *see* Central Sydney Area Health Service.
Daldt, B.W. 1981. 'Anger: An Alienation Communication Hazard for Nurses', *Nursing Outlook*, 29, pp 213–45.
Gournay, K. 2001, *The Recognition, Prevention and Therapeutic Management of Violence in Mental Health Care: A Consultation Document*, United Kingdom Central Council for Nursing, Midwifery and Health Visiting, London.
Jackson, D., Clare, J. & Mannix, J. 2002, 'Who Would Want to Be a Nurse? Violence in the Workplace—a Factor in Recruitment and Retention', *Journal of Nursing Management*, 10 (1), pp 13–20.
New South Wales Health Department 2001, *Management of Adults with Severe Behavioural Disturbances*, Author, Sydney.
NSWHD, *see* New South Wales Health Department.
RCPsych, *see* Royal College of Psychiatrists.
Royal College of Psychiatrists Special Working Party on Clinical Assessment and Management of Risk 1996, *Assessment and Clinical Management of Risk of Harm to Other People*, Author, London.
Smeltzer, S.C. & Bare, B.G. 2000, *Brunner & Suddarth's Textbook of Medical–Surgical Nursing*, 9th edn, Lippincott ,Williams & Wilkins, Philadelphia.
Tonge, B. 1998, 'Intellectual Disability and Mental Health: a Neglected Issue of Major Importance', *AusEinetter*, Issue 4, <http://auseinet.flinders.edu.au/netter4/netter02.htm>.
Turnbull, J. & Paterson, B. (eds) 1999, *Aggression and Violence: Approaches to Effective Management*, Macmillan, London.
Volkmar, F.R. 2001, 'Review of Psychiatric and Behavioural Disorders in Developmental Disabilities and Mental Retardation', N. Bouras (ed.), *American Journal of Psychiatry*, vol. 158 (3), p. 513.
Whittingdon, R. 2002, 'Attitudes Towards Patient Aggression Amongst Mental Health Nurses in the 'Zero Tolerance' Era: Associations with Burnout and Length of Experience', *Journal of Clinical Nursing*, 11 (6), pp 819–25.

Chapter 22 Evidence-based Management

Buerhaus, P.I. 1998, 'Creating a New Place in a Competitive Market: The Value of Nursing Care', in Hein, E.C. (ed.), *Contemporary Leadership Behaviour*, 5th edn, Lippincott.
Carr, W. & Kemis, S. 1986, *Becoming Critical: Education, Knowledge and Action Research*, Farmer Press, Lewes.
Delbecq, A.L., Van de Ven, H. & Gustafson, D.H., 1975, *Group Techniques for Programme Planning: A Guide to Nominal Group and Delphi Processes*, Scott-Foresman, Glenview, Illinois.
French, P. 1994, 'An Experimental Study of the Effects of Learning Climate on Patient-Centred Decision-Making', *International Journal of Nursing Studies*, 31(6) pp 593–605.
French, P. 2000, 'Evidence-based Nursing: A Change Dynamic in Managed Care System', *Journal of Nursing Management*, 8, 141–7.
French, P. 2002, 'What is the Evidence on Evidence-Based Nursing? An Epistemological Concern', *Journal of Advanced Nursing*, 37(3),250–7.
French, P., Ho, M. & Lee, T. 2002, 'A Delphi Survey of Evidence-based Nursing Practice Research Priorities in Hong Kong', *Journal of Nursing Management*, 10, 265–73.
Ganong, L.H. 1987, 'Integrative Reviews on Nursing Research', *Research in Nursing and Health*, 10(1): 1–11.

Gelatt, H.B. 1962, 'Decision-Making: A Conceptual Frame of Reference for Counselling', *Journal of Counselling Psychology*, 9(3), 240–5.

Gray, J.A.M. 1997, *Evidence-based Health Care: How to Make Health Policy and Management Decisions*, Churchill Livingstone, New York.

Greenwood, J. 1996, 'Nursing Theories: An Introduction to their Development and Application', in *Nursing Theory in Australia: Development and Application*, Greenwood, J. (ed.), Addison-Wesley, Melbourne.

Jackson, G.B. 1980, 'Methods for Integrating Reviews', *Review of Educational Research*, 50, 428–60.

Lewin, K. 1947, 'Frontiers in Group Dynamics: Social Planning and Group Dynamics', *Human Relations*, 1 (1), 143–52.

Linstone, H.A. & Turoff, M. 1975, *The Delphi Method: Techniques and Applications*, Addison Wesley, Reading.

Lussier, R.N. 2003, *Management Fundamentals: Concepts, Applications, Skills, Development*, 2nd edn, Thompson, Cincinnati.

Matthews, P. 2002, 'Case Management Information Systems: How To Put the Pieces Together Now and beyond Year 2000', *Lippincott's Case Management*, 7(6): 255–60.

Plunkett, W.R., Attner, R.F. & Allen, G.S. 2002, *Management: Meeting and Exceeding Customer Expectations*, 7th edn, Thompson, Cincinnati.

Index

motivation (*continued*)
  strategies of transformational leadership
    40–3
  theories of leadership 38–40
  transactional leadership 38, 39
  transformational leadership 38–9
multidisciplinary teams *see*
    interdisciplinary relations

nurse manager as educator *see* education
nurse manager, role of *see* individual
    subject entries
nursing, definition of 31
nursing research *see* research
nursing shortage 94, 163, 174, 175, 176,
    178, 209, 223

occupational health and safety 117–27
  see also quality management; risk
    management
  auditing 124, 125
  benefits of 127
  bullying *see* bullying
  communication 124–5
  complaints 126
  competence 124, 125
  consultation and cooperation 124
  contractors 120, 121
  costs 119
  documentation and record-keeping
    124–5
  duty of care 118
  employers and 117, 118, 122
  environmental hazards 118
  equipment and products 123
  ergonomic hazards 117, 118, 122
  fatigue 117, 126
  hazards and risks 118–27
  human resources 121, 122
  infectious diseases 117, 118
  information 121, 122
  inputs 120–2
  legal requirements 118
  model for 120
  outputs 126–7
  physical resources 120–1, 122
  physical work environment 118, 123
  policies and procedures 146
  probability and severity 118

occupational health and safety (*continued*)
  radiation 117
  reporting 119
  risk control and management 120–7
  risks and hazards 118–27
  rostering and 117, 118, 126
  safe work procedures 123–4
  safety management system 124–6
  security 124, 126
  supervision 124
  toxic drugs and chemicals 117, 118
  violence 117, 126
  work activities 117, 119, 123–6

patient liaison officers 113, 254
performance management 93–104
  see also job descriptions; policies and
    procedures; recruiting
  conducting performance reviews 96–103
  confidentiality and 95, 97, 98
  counselling and 72, 97, 98, 101, 104
  discipline and 94, 101
  documentation of 99, 100–1
  education and 94
  environment for 98
  feedback 95, 97, 98, 99, 100, 102, 103
  frequency of 96–7
  importance of 94–5
  job descriptions and 96, 99, 153, 155,
    156, 160, 161
  key performance indicators 102, 103
  key points in 99
  mentoring and 94, 97, 99, 102, 103
  motivation and 93, 96
  policies and procedures 104
  poor performance and disagreements
    103–4
  positives and negatives of 95–6
  preparation for 99
  research role and 102
  respect and 8
  risk management and 109
  role clarification 96
  skills required for 100
  staff retention and 94
  style of 93, 99–100
  supports 97, 101–2, 103, 104
  terminology 93
  timing of 97

From the extensive list of books from Ausmed Publications, the publisher especially recommends the following as being of interest to readers of *Nurse Managers: A Guide to Practice*.
All of these titles are available from the publisher: Ausmed Publications, 277 Mt Alexander Road, Ascot Vale, Melbourne, Victoria 3032, Australia
website: <www.ausmed.com.au>; email: <ausmed@ausmed.com.au>

Aged Care Nursing: A Guide to Practice
Edited by Susan Carmody and Sue Forster

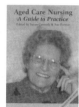

The aged population has grown markedly throughout the world, but there is a shortage of experienced nurses with expertise in the holistic care of the elderly. This book is written to inspire and empower such nurses. *Aged Care Nursing: A Guide to Practice* is written by clinicians for clinicians. The inclusion of evidence-based and outcome-based practices throughout the book ensures that all readers, be they novices or experts, will have a reliable and comprehensive reference to guide their practice.
Each author is a recognised expert in his or her subject area, and all present their topics with a focus that is practical, rather than academic. Available as textbook alone or as audiobook–textbook package.

Palliative Care Nursing: A Guide to Practice (2nd edn)
Edited by Margaret O'Connor and Sanchia Aranda

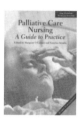

This second edition of Palliative Care Nursing has been totally revised, rewritten, and redesigned. The result is a comprehensive handsome volume that builds upon the successful formula of the popular first edition. All nurses and other health professionals with an interest in this vital subject will welcome this new edition as an essential addition to their libraries. This is the definitive textbook on palliative-care nursing.

Evidence-based Management: A practical guide for health professionals
Rosemary Stewart

There are two dominant themes in modern nursing. The first is evidence-based practice. The second is modern management theory. This book brings these two themes together in a fascinating study of evidence-based management. *Evidence-based Management* is presented with a clear layout, illustrative cases studies, and a pragmatic approach to the practicalities and problems of modern management. This book is an essential guide for health managers and clinicians who have managerial responsibilities in a variety of public and private settings. Not for sale outside Australia and New Zealand.

From the extensive list of books from Ausmed Publications, the publisher especially recommends the following as being of interest to readers of *Nurse Managers: A Guide to Practice*.

All of these titles are available from the publisher: Ausmed Publications, 277 Mt Alexander Road, Ascot Vale, Melbourne, Victoria 3032, Australia

website: <www.ausmed.com.au>; email: <ausmed@ausmed.com.au>

Dementia Nursing: A Guide to Practice
Edited by Rosalie Hudson

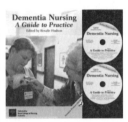

Dementia is one of the major health problems of our ageing society and dementia nursing is one of the most important and highly skilled of nursing specialities. As another volume in Ausmed's growing 'Guide to Practice' series, this is the definitive textbook on dementia nursing. The chapters are written primarily by nurses for nurses. But dementia nursing is essentially an exercise in teamwork, and valuable contributions and insights are offered by other health professionals, carers, artists, and relatives from a variety of backgrounds and countries. The result is a comprehensive international volume on all aspects of dementia nursing. Available as textbook alone or as audiobook–textbook package.

Assertiveness and the Manager's Job
Annie Phillips

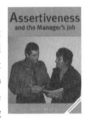

Assertiveness is often equated with selfishness, aggression, or a lack of humour. But true assertiveness is not negative. True assertiveness is positive, creative, and empowering. The first part of *Assertiveness and the Manager's Job* describes what assertiveness is and teaches some of the skills needed to become assertive—how to deal with requests, anger, conflict, and criticism. In the second part of this book, these learned skills are applied to common work situations—managing people, setting goals, and facilitating change by using assertiveness effectively. This book was primarily directed to general practitioners practice in the UK health system. However, the principles and practices described here are applicable to healthcare managers in a variety of professions all over the world. In particular, nurse managers, the majority of whom are women, will find this book to be an invaluable resource in acquiring the skills of caring and creative assertiveness in the workplace. Not for sale outside Australia and New Zealand.

Communication and the Manager's Job
Annie Phillips

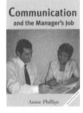

Good communication is essential to good management. Good communication allows those in positions of leadership to understand others, solve problems, manage conflict, and develop new personal managerial skills. Good managers are good communicators. The aim of *Communication and the Manager's Job* is to enhance the interpersonal communication skills of healthcare managers so that they become more effective listeners, understand their colleagues, and respond skilfully and sensitively to the many challenges presented by modern healthcare management. Although primarily written for general practice managers in the UK, the book has universal applicability and appeal to nurse managers, other healthcare managers, and all members of the health team who have an interest in their own personal and professional development. Not for sale outside Australia and New Zealand.